STATISTICS AT SQUARE ONE

STATISTICS AT SQUARE ONE

NINTH EDITION

T D V SWINSCOW

Revised by
M J CAMPBELL
University of Southampton

BMJ
Publishing
Group

First edition 1976
Second edition 1977
Third edition 1978
Fourth edition 1978
Fifth edition 1979
Sixth edition 1980
Seventh edition 1980
Eighth edition 1983

First published in 1976
by the BMJ Publishing Group, BMA House, Tavistock Square, London WC1H 9JR

British Library Cataloguing in Publication Data

A catalogue record for this book is available from the British Library

ISBN 0-7279-0916-9

Printed and bound in Great Britain by Latimer Trend & Company Ltd., Plymouth

Contents

To my father

Preface

It is with trepidation that one rewrites a best seller, and Dougal Swinscow's *Statistics at Square One* was one of the best selling statistical text books in the UK. It is difficult to decide how much to alter without destroying the quality that proved so popular. I chose to retain the format and structure of the original book. Most of the original examples remain; they are realistic, if not real, and tracking down the original sources to provide references would be impossible. However, I have removed the chromatic pseudonyms of the investigators. All new examples utilise real data, the source of which is referenced.

Much has changed in medical statistics since the original edition was published in 1976. Desktop computers now provide statistical facilities unimaginable then, even for mainframe enthusiasts. I think the main change has been an emphasis now on looking and plotting the data first, and on estimation rather than simple hypothesis testing. I have tried to reflect these changes in the new edition. I have found it a useful pedagogic device to pose questions to the students, and so have incorporated questions commonly asked by students or consultees at the end of each chapter. These questions cover issues often not explicitly addressed in elementary text books, such as how far one should test assumptions before proceeding with statistical tests.

I have included a number of new techniques, such as stem and leaf plots, box whisker plots, data transformation, the χ^2 test for trend and t test with unequal variance. I have also included a chapter on survival analysis, with the Kaplan–Meier survival curve and the log rank test, as these are now in common use. I have replaced the Kendall rank correlation coefficient by the Spearman; in spite of the theoretical advantages of the former, most statistical packages compute only the latter. The section on linear regression has been extended. I have added a final chapter on the design of studies, and would make a plea for it not to be ignored. Studies rarely fail for want of a significance test, but a flawed design may be fatal. To keep the book short I have removed some details of hand calculation.

I have assumed that the reader will not want to master a complicated statistical program, but has available a simple scientific calculator, which should cost about the same as this book. However, no serious statistical analysis should be undertaken these days without a computer. There are many good and inexpensive statistical programs. Of these Epi-Info, which is produced by the Center for Disease Control (CDC) Atlanta and the World Health Organization (WHO) in Geneva is available free over our World Wide Web Server (http://medstats.soton.ac.uk). Another useful program is CIA (Confidence Interval Analysis) which is available from the *BMJ*.

I am most grateful to Tina Perry for secretarial help, to Simon Child for producing the figures, and to Simon Child and Jide Olayinka for help with word processing. I am particularly grateful to Paul Little, Steven Julious, Ruth Pickering and David Coggon who commented on all or part of the book, and who made many suggestions for improvement. Any errors remain my own. Finally, thanks to Deborah Reece of the *BMJ* who asked me to revise the book and was patient with the delays.

M J Campbell
August 1995

1 Data display and summary

Types of data

The first step, before any calculations or plotting of data, is to decide what type of data one is dealing with. There are a number of typologies, but one that has proven useful is given in Table 1.1.

The basic distinction is between *quantitative* variables (for which one asks "how much?") and *categorical* variables (for which one asks "what type?").

Quantitative variables can be *continuous* or *discrete*. Continuous variables, such as height, can in theory take any value within a given range. Examples of discrete variables are: number of children in a family, number of attacks of asthma per week.

Categorical variables are either *nominal* (unordered) or *ordinal* (ordered). Examples of nominal variables are male/female, alive/ dead, blood group O, A, B, AB. For nominal variables with more than two categories the order does not matter. For example, one cannot say that people in blood group B lie between those in A and those in AB. Sometimes, however, people can provide ordered responses, such as grade of breast cancer, or they can "agree", "neither agree nor disagree", or "disagree" with some statement. In this case the order does matter and it is usually important to account for it.

1

Table 1.1   *Examples of types of data*

	Quantitative
Continuous	Discrete
Blood pressure, height, weight, age	Number of children Number of attacks of asthma per week

	Categorical
Ordinal (Ordered categories)	Nominal (Unordered categories)
Grade of breast cancer Better, same, worse Disagree, neutral, agree	Sex (male/female) Alive or dead Blood group O, A, B, AB

Variables shown at the left of Table 1.1 can be converted to ones further to the right by using "cut off points". For example, blood pressure can be turned into a nominal variable by defining "hypertension" as a diastolic blood pressure greater than 90 mmHg, and "normotension" as blood pressure less than or equal to 90 mmHg. Height (continuous) can be converted into "short", "average" or "tall" (ordinal).

In general it is easier to summarise categorical variables, and so quantitative variables are often converted to categorical ones for descriptive purposes. To make a clinical decision on someone, one does not need to know the exact serum potassium level (continuous) but whether it is within the normal range (nominal). It may be easier to think of the proportion of the population who are hypertensive than the distribution of blood pressure. However, categorising a continuous variable reduces the amount of information available and statistical tests will in general be more sensitive—that is they will have more power (see Chapter 5 for a definition of *power*) for a continuous variable than the corresponding nominal one, although more assumptions may have to be made about the data. Categorising data is therefore useful for summarising results, but not for statistical analysis. It is often not appreciated that the choice of appropriate cut off points can be difficult, and different choices can lead to different conclusions about a set of data.

These definitions of types of data are not unique, nor are they mutually exclusive, and are given as an aid to help an investigator decide how to display and analyse data. One should not debate overlong the typology of a particular variable!

Stem and leaf plots

Before any statistical calculation, even the simplest, is performed the data should be tabulated or plotted. If they are quantitative and relatively few, say up to about 30, they are conveniently written down in order of size.

For example, a paediatric registrar in a district general hospital is investigating the amount of lead in the urine of children from a nearby housing estate. In a particular street there are 15 children whose ages range from 1 year to under 16, and in a preliminary study the registrar has found the following amounts of urinary lead (in μmol/24 h), given in Table 1.2 in what is called an *array*:

Table 1.2   *Urinary concentration of lead in 15 children from housing estate (μmol/24 h)*

0·6,   2·6,   0·1,   1·1,   0·4,   2·0,   0·8,   1·3,   1·2,   1·5,   3·2,   1·7,   1·9,   1·9,   2·2

A simple way to order, and also to display, the data is to use a stem and leaf plot. To do this we need to abbreviate the observations to two significant digits. In the case of the urinary concentration data, the digit to the left of the decimal point is the "stem" and the digit to the right the "leaf".

We first write the stems in order down the page. We then work along the data set, writing the leaves down "as they come". Thus, for the first data point, we write a 6 opposite the 0 stem. These are as given in Figure 1.1.

```
Stem    Leaf
0       6   1   4   8
1       1   3   2   5   7   9   9
2       6   0   2
3       2
```

Figure 1.1   Stem and leaf "as they come".

We then order the leaves, as in Figure 1.2.

Stem	Leaf						
0	1	4	6	8			
1	1	2	3	5	7	9	9
2	0	2	6				
3	2						

Figure 1.2   Ordered stem and leaf plot.

The advantage of first setting the figures out in order of size and not simply feeding them straight from notes into a calculator (for example, to find their mean) is that the relation of each to the next can be looked at. Is there a steady progression, a noteworthy hump, a considerable gap? Simple inspection can disclose irregularities. Furthermore, a glance at the figures gives information on their *range*. The smallest value is 0·1 and the largest is 3·2 μmol/24 h.

Median

To find the median (or mid point) we need to identify the point which has the property that half the data are greater than it, and half the data are less than it. For 15 points, the mid point is clearly the eighth largest, so that seven points are less than the median, and seven points are greater than it. This is easily obtained from Figure 1.2 by counting the eighth leaf, which is 1·5 μmol/24 h.

To find the median for an even number of points, the procedure is as follows. Suppose the paediatric registrar obtained a further set of 16 urinary lead concentrations from children living in the countryside in the same county as the hospital (Table 1.3).

Table 1.3   Urinary concentration of lead in 16 rural children μmol/24 h

0·2, 0·3, 0·6, 0·7, 0·8, 1·5, 1·7, 1·8, 1·9, 1·9, 2·0, 2·0, 2·1, 2·8, 3·1, 3·4

To obtain the median we average the eighth and ninth points (1·8 and 1·9) to get 1·85 μmol/24 h. In general, if n is even, we average the n/2th largest and the n/2 + 1th largest observations.

The main advantage of using the median as a measure of location is that it is "robust" to outliers. For example, if we had accidentally written 34 rather than 3·4 in Table 1.2, the median would still have been 1·85. One disadvantage is that it is tedious to order a large number of observations by hand (there is usually no "median" button on a calculator).

Measures of variation

It is informative to have some measure of the variation of observations about the median. The range is very susceptible to what are known as *outliers*, points well outside the main body of the data. For example, if we had made the mistake of writing 34 instead 3·4 in Table 1.2, then the range would be written as 0·1 to 34 μmol/24 h, which is clearly misleading.

A more robust approach is to divide the distribution of the data into four, and find the points below which are 25%, 50% and 75% of the distribution. These are known as *quartiles*, and the median is the second quartile. The variation of the data can be summarised in the interquartile range, the distance between the first and third quartile. With small data sets and if the sample size is not divisible by four, it may not be possible to divide the data set into exact quarters, and there are a variety of proposed methods to estimate the quartiles. A simple, consistent method is to find the points midway between each end of the range and the median. Thus, from Figure 1.2, there are eight points between and including the smallest, 0·1, and the median, 1·5. Thus the mid point lies between 0·8 and 1·1, or 0·95. This is the first quartile. Similarly the third quartile is mid way between 1·9 and 2·0, or 1·95. Thus, the interquartile range is 0·95 to 1·95 μmol/24 h.

Data display

The simplest way to show data is a dot plot. Figure 1.3 shows the data from Tables 1.2 and 1.3 together with the median for each set.

Sometimes the points in separate plots may be linked in some way, for example the data in Tables 1.2 and 1.3 may result from a matched case control study (see Chapter 13 for a description of this type of study) in which individuals from the countryside were matched by age and sex with individuals from the town. If possible

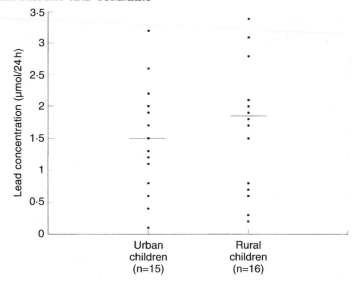

Figure 1.3   Dot plot of urinary lead concentrations for urban and rural children.

the links should be maintained in the display, for example by joining matching individuals in Figure 1.3. This can lead to a more sensitive way of examining the data.

When the data sets are large, plotting individual points can be cumbersome. An alternative is a box–whisker plot. The box is marked by the first and third quartile, and the whiskers extend to the range. The median is also marked in the box, as shown in Figure 1.4.

It is easy to include more information in a box–whisker plot. One method, which is implemented in some computer programs, is to extend the whiskers only to points that are 1·5 times the interquartile range below the first quartile or above the third quartile, and to show remaining points as dots, so that the number of outlying points is shown.

Histograms

Suppose the paediatric registrar referred to earlier extends the urban study to the entire estate in which the children live. He

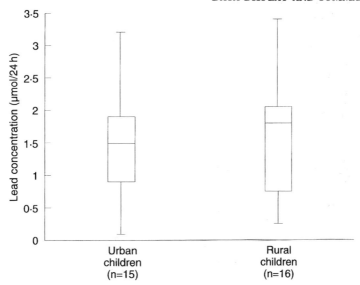

Figure 1.4   Box–whisker plot of data from Figure 1.3.

Table 1.4   Lead concentration in 140 urban children

Lead concentration (μmol/24 h)	Number of children
0–	2
0·4–	7
0·8–	10
1·2–	16
1·6–	23
2·0–	28
2·4–	19
2·8–	16
3·2–	11
3·6–	7
4·0–	1
4·4	
Total	140

obtains figures for the urinary lead concentration in 140 children aged over 1 year and under 16. We can display these data as a grouped frequency table (Table 1.4).

These can also be displayed as a histogram as in Figure 1.5.

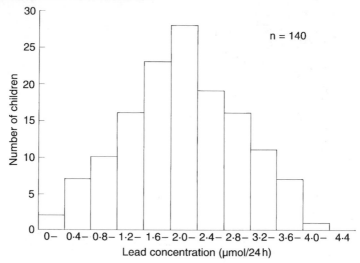

Figure 1.5   Histogram of data from Table 1.4.

Bar charts

Suppose, of the 140 children, 20 lived in owner occupied houses, 70 lived in council houses and 50 lived in private rented accommodation. Figures from the census suggest that for this age group, throughout the county, 50% live in owner occupied houses, 30% in council houses, and 20% in private rented accommodation. Type of accommodation is a categorical variable, which can be displayed in a bar chart. We first express our data as percentages: 14% owner occupied, 50% council house, 36% private rented. We then display the data as a bar chart. The sample size should always be given (Figure 1.6).

Common questions

How many groups should I have for a histogram?

In general one should choose enough groups to show the shape of a distribution, but not too many to lose the shape in the noise. It is partly aesthetic judgement but, in general, between 5 and 15, depending on the sample size, gives a reasonable picture. Try to keep the intervals (known also as "bin widths") equal. With equal intervals the height of the bars and the area of the bars are both

8

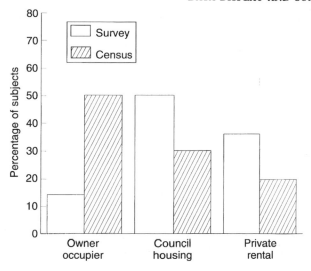

Figure 1.6   Bar chart of housing data for 140 children and comparable census data.

proportional to the number of subjects in the group. With unequal intervals this link is lost, and interpretation of the figure can be difficult.

What is the distinction between a histogram and a bar chart?

Alas, with modern graphics programs the distinction is often lost. A *histogram* shows the distribution of a continuous variable and, since the variable is continuous, there should be no gaps between the bars. A *bar chart* shows the distribution of a discrete variable or a categorical one, and so will have spaces between the bars. It is a mistake to use a bar chart to display a summary statistic such as a mean, particularly when it is accompanied by some measure of variation to produce a "dynamite plunger plot".[1] It is better to use a box–whisker plot.

What is the best way to display data?

The general principle should be, as far as possible, to show the original data and to try not to obscure the design of a study in the display. Within the constraints of legibility show as much information as possible. If data points are matched or from the

9

same patients link them with lines.[2] When displaying the relationship between two quantitative variables, use a scatter plot (Chapter 11) in preference to categorising one or both of the variables.

1 Campbell MJ. How to present numerical results. In: *How to do it*: 2. London: BMJ Publishing, 1995:77–83.
2 Matthews JNS, Altman DG, Campbell MJ, Royston JP. Analysis of serial measurements in medical research. *BMJ* 1990;**300**:230–5.

Exercises

Exercise 1.1

From the 140 children whose urinary concentration of lead were investigated 40 were chosen who were aged at least 1 year but under 5 years. The following concentrations of copper (in μmol/24 h) were found.

0·70, 0·45, 0·72, 0·30, 1·16, 0·69, 0·83, 0·74, 1·24, 0·77,
0·65, 0·76, 0·42, 0·94, 0·36, 0·98, 0·64, 0·90, 0·63, 0·55,
0·78, 0·10, 0·52, 0·42, 0·58, 0·62, 1·12, 0·86, 0·74, 1·04,
0·65, 0·66, 0·81, 0·48, 0·85, 0·75, 0·73, 0·50, 0·34, 0·88

Find the median, range and quartiles.

2 Mean and standard deviation

The median is known as a measure of location; that is, it tells us where the data are. As stated in Chapter 1, we do not need to know all the exact values to calculate the median; if we made the smallest value even smaller or the largest value even larger, it would not change the value of the median. Thus the median does not use all the information in the data and so it can be shown to be less efficient than the mean or average, which does use all values of the data. To calculate the mean we add up the observed values and divide by the number of them. The total of the values obtained in Table 1.1 was $22.5\ \mu mol/24\,h$, which was divided by their number, 15, to give a mean of $1.5\ \mu mol/24\,h$. This familiar process is conveniently expressed by the following symbols:

$$\bar{x} = \frac{(\Sigma x)}{n}.$$

$\bar{x}$ (pronounced "x bar") signifies the mean; x is each of the values of urinary lead; n is the number of these values; and Σ, the Greek capital sigma (our "S") denotes "sum of". A major disadvantage of the mean is that it is sensitive to outlying points. For example, replacing 2.2 by 22 in Table 1.1 increases the mean to $2.82\ \mu mol/24\,h$, whereas the median will be unchanged.

As well as measures of location we need measures of how variable the data are. We met two of these measures, the range and interquartile range, in Chapter 1.

The range is an important measurement, for figures at the top and bottom of it denote the findings furthest removed from the generality. However, they do not give much indication of the spread of observations about the mean. This is where the standard deviation (SD) comes in.

The theoretical basis of the standard deviation is complex and need not trouble the ordinary user. We will discuss sampling and populations in Chapter 3. A practical point to note here is that, when the population from which the data arise have a distribution that is approximately "Normal" (or Gaussian), then the standard deviation provides a useful basis for interpreting the data in terms of probability.

The Normal distribution is represented by a family of curves defined uniquely by two parameters, which are the mean and the standard deviation of the population. The curves are always symmetrically bell shaped, but the extent to which the bell is compressed or flattened out depends on the standard deviation of the population. However, the mere fact that a curve is bell shaped does not mean that it represents a Normal distribution, because other distributions may have a similar sort of shape.

Many biological characteristics conform to a Normal distribution closely enough for it to be commonly used—for example, heights of adult men and women, blood pressures in a healthy population, random errors in many types of laboratory measurements and biochemical data. Figure 2.1 shows a Normal curve calculated from the diastolic blood pressures of 500 men, mean 82 mmHg, standard deviation 10 mmHg. The ranges representing ± 1 SD, ± 2 SD, and ± 3 SD about the mean are marked. A more extensive set of values is given in Table A in the Appendix.

The reason why the standard deviation is such a useful measure of the scatter of the observations is this: if the observations follow a Normal distribution, a range covered by one standard deviation above the mean and one standard deviation below it ($\bar{x} \pm 1$ SD) includes about 68% of the observations; a range of two standard deviations above and two below ($\bar{x} \pm 2$ SD) about 95% of the observations; and of three standard deviations above and three below ($\bar{x} \pm 3$ SD) about 99·7% of the observations. Consequently,

12

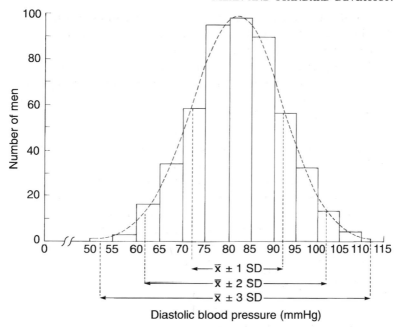

Figure 2.1 *Normal curve calculated from diastolic blood pressures of 500 men, mean 82 mmHg, standard deviation 10 mmHg.*

if we know the mean and standard deviation of a set of observations, we can obtain some useful information by simple arithmetic. By putting one, two, or three standard deviations above and below the mean we can estimate the ranges that would be expected to include about 68%, 95%, and 99·7% of the observations.

Standard deviation from ungrouped data

The standard deviation is a summary measure of the differences of each observation from the mean. If the differences themselves were added up, the positive would exactly balance the negative and so their sum would be zero. Consequently the squares of the differences are added. The sum of the squares is then divided by the number of observations *minus one* to give the mean of the squares, and the square root is taken to bring the measurements back to the units we started with. (The division by the number of observations *minus one* instead of the number of observations itself

13

to obtain the mean square is because "degrees of freedom" must be used. In these circumstances they are one less than the total. The theoretical justification for this need not trouble the user in practice.)

To gain an intuitive feel for degrees of freedom, consider choosing a chocolate from a box of n chocolates. Every time we come to choose a chocolate we have a choice, until we come to the last one (normally one with a nut in it!), and then we have no choice. Thus we have n–1 choices, or "degrees of freedom".

The calculation of the variance is illustrated in Table 2.1 with the 15 readings in the preliminary study of urinary lead concentrations (Table 1.1). The readings are set out in column (1). In column (2) the difference between each reading and the mean is recorded. The sum of the differences is 0. In column (3) the differences are squared, and the sum of those squares is given at the bottom of the column.

Table 2.1   Calculation of standard deviation

(1) Lead concentration (μmol/24 h) x	(2) Differences from mean $x - \bar{x}$	(3) Differences squared $(x - \bar{x})^2$	(4) Observations in col (1) squared x^2
0·1	−1·4	1·96	0·01
0·4	−1·1	1·21	0·16
0·6	−0·9	0·81	0·36
0·8	−0·7	0·49	0·64
1·1	−0·4	0·16	1·21
1·2	−0·3	0·09	1·44
1·3	−0·2	0·04	1·69
1·5	0	0	2·25
1·7	0·2	0·04	2·89
1·9	0·4	0·16	3·61
1·9	0·4	0·16	3·61
2·0	0·5	0·25	4·00
2·2	0·7	0·49	4·84
2·6	1·1	1·21	6·76
3·2	1·7	2·89	10·24
Total 22·5	0	9·96	43·71

n = 15, $\bar{x}$ = 1·5.

The sum of the squares of the differences (or deviations) from the mean, 9·96, is now divided by the total number of observations

14

minus one, to give the *variance*. Thus,

$$\text{Variance} = \frac{\Sigma(x - \bar{x})^2}{n-1}.$$

In this case we find:

$$\text{Variance} = \frac{9 \cdot 96}{14} = 0 \cdot 7114 \ (\mu\text{mol}/24\,\text{h})^2.$$

Finally, the square root of the variance provides the standard deviation:

$$\text{SD} = \sqrt{\frac{\Sigma(x - \bar{x})^2}{n-1}}$$

from which we get

$$\text{SD} = \sqrt{0 \cdot 7114} = 0 \cdot 843 \ \mu\text{mol}/24\,\text{h}.$$

This procedure illustrates the structure of the standard deviation, in particular that the two extreme values 0·1 and 3·2 contribute most to the sum of the differences squared.

Calculator procedure

Most inexpensive calculators have procedures that enable one to calculate the mean and standard deviations directly, using the "SD" mode. For example, on modern Casio calculators one presses **SHIFT** and '·' and a little "SD" symbol should appear on the display. On earlier Casios one presses **INV** and **MODE**, whereas on a Sharp **2nd F** and **Stat** should be used. The data are stored via the **M+** button. Thus, having set the calculator into the "SD" or "Stat" mode, from Table 2.1 we enter 0·1 **M+**, 0·4 **M+**, etc. When all the data are entered, we can check that the correct number of observations have been included by **Shift** and **n** and "15" should be displayed. The mean is displayed by **Shift** and $\bar{x}$ and the standard deviation by **Shift** and σ_{n-1}. Avoid pressing **Shift** and **AC** between these operations as this clears the statistical memory. There is another button (σ_n) on many calculators. This uses the divisor n rather than n − 1 in the calculation of the standard deviation. On a Sharp calculator σ_n is denoted σ, whereas σ_{n-1} is denoted s. These are the "population" values, and are derived assuming that an entire population is available or that interest focuses solely on the data in hand, and the results are not going to be generalised (see Chapter 3 for details of samples and populations). As this situation very rarely arises, σ_{n-1} should be used and σ_n ignored, although even for moderate sample sizes the difference is going to be small. Remember to return to normal mode before resuming calculations because many of the usual functions are not available in "Stat" mode. On a modern Casio this is **Shift 0**. On earlier Casios and on Sharps one repeats the sequence that call up the "Stat" mode. Some calculators stay in "Stat" mode even when switched off.

Mullee[1] provides advice on choosing and using a calculator.

The calculator formulas use the relationship

$$\sigma^2{}_n = \frac{1}{n}\Sigma(x-\bar{x})^2 = \frac{1}{n}\left[\Sigma x^2 - \frac{(\Sigma x)^2}{n}\right] = \frac{\Sigma x^2}{n} - \bar{x}^2.$$

The right hand expression can be easily memorised by the expression "mean of the squares minus the mean square". The sample variance $\sigma^2{}_{n-1}$ is obtained from $\sigma^2{}_{n-1} = n\sigma^2{}_n/(n-1)$.

The above equation can be seen to be true in Table 2.1, where the sum of the square of the observations, Σx^2, is given as 43·71. We thus obtain

$$(43\cdot71)^2 - \frac{(22\cdot5)^2}{15} = 9\cdot96$$

the same value given for the total in column (3). Care should be taken because this formula involves subtracting two large numbers to get a small one, and can lead to incorrect results if the numbers are very large. For example, try finding the standard deviation of 100001, 100002, 100003 on a calculator. The correct answer is 1, but many calculators will give 0 because of rounding error. The solution is to subtract a large number from each of the observations (say 100000) and calculate the standard deviation on the remainders, namely 1, 2 and 3.

16

Standard deviation from grouped data

We can also calculate a standard deviation for discrete quantitative variables. For example, in addition to studying the lead concentration in the urine of 140 children, the paediatrician asked how often each of them had been examined by a doctor during the year. After collecting the information he tabulated the data shown in Table 2.2, columns (1) and (2). The mean is calculated by multiplying column (1) by column (2), adding the products, and dividing by the total number of observations.

Table 2.2 *Calculation of the standard deviation from qualitative discrete data*

(1) Number of visits to or by doctor	(2) Number of children	(3) Col (2) × Col (1)	(4) Col (1) squared	(5) Col (2) × Col (4)
0	2	0	0	0
1	8	8	1	8
2	27	54	4	108
3	45	135	9	405
4	38	152	16	608
5	15	75	25	375
6	4	24	36	144
7	1	7	49	49
Total	140	455		1697

Mean number of visits $= 455/140 = 3.25$.

As we did for continuous data, to calculate the standard deviation we square each of the observations in turn. In this case the observation is the number of visits, but because we have several children in each class, shown in column (2), each squared number (column (4)), must be multiplied by the number of children. The sum of squares is given at the foot of column (5), namely 1697. We then use the calculator formula to find the variance:

$$\text{Variance} = \frac{(1697 - 455^2/140)}{139} = 1.57$$

17

and

$$SD = \sqrt{1\cdot57} = 1\cdot25.$$

Note that although the number of visits is not Normally distributed, the distribution is reasonably symmetrical about the mean. The approximate 95% range is given by

$$3\cdot25 - 2 \times 1\cdot25 = 0\cdot75 \text{ to } 3\cdot25 + 2 \times 1\cdot25 = 5\cdot75.$$

This excludes two children with no visits and six children with six or more visits. Thus there are eight of $140 = 5\cdot7\%$ outside the theoretical 95% range.

Note that it is common for discrete quantitative variables to have what is known as *skewed* distributions, that is they are not symmetrical. One clue to lack of symmetry from derived statistics is when the mean and the median differ considerably. Another is when the standard deviation is of the same order of magnitude as the mean, but the observations must be non-negative. Sometimes a transformation will convert a skewed distribution into a symmetrical one. When the data are counts, such as number of visits to a doctor, often the square root transformation will help, and if there are no zero or negative values a logarithmic transformation will render the distribution more symmetrical.

Data transformation

An anaesthetist measures the pain of a procedure using a 100 mm visual analogue scale on seven patients. The results are given in Table 2.3, together with the $\log_e$ transformation (the **ln** button on a calculator).

Table 2.3 Results from pain score on seven patients (mm)

| Original scale: | 1, | 1, | 2, | 3, | 3, | 6, | 56 |
| Log$_e$ scale: | 0, | 0, | 0·69, | 1·10, | 1·10, | 1·79, | 4·03 |

The data are plotted in Figure 2.2, which shows that the outlier does not appear so extreme in the logged data. The mean and median are 10·29 and 2, respectively, for the original data, with a standard deviation of 20·22. Where the mean is

18

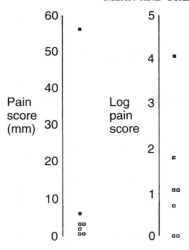

Figure 2.2   Dot plots of original and logged data from pain scores.

bigger than the median, the distribution is positively skewed. For the logged data the mean and median are 1·24 and 1·10 respectively, indicating that the logged data have a more symmetrical distribution. Thus it would be better to analyse the logged transformed data in statistical tests than using the original scale.

In reporting these results, the median of the raw data would be given, but it should be explained that the statistical test wascarried out on the transformed data. Note that the median of the logged data is the same as the log of the median of the raw data—however, this is not true for the mean. The mean of the logged data is not necessarily equal to the log of the mean of the raw data. The antilog (**exp** or e^x on a calculator) of the mean of the logged data is known as the *geometric mean*, and is often a better summary statistic than the mean for data from positively skewed distributions. For these data the geometric mean in 3·45 mm.

Between subjects and within subjects standard deviation

If repeated measurements are made of, say, blood pressure on an individual, these measurements are likely to vary. This is

19

within subject, or intrasubject, variability and we can calculate a standard deviation of these observations. If the observations are close together in time, this standard deviation is often described as the *measurement error*. Measurements made on different subjects vary according to between subject, or intersubject, variability. If many observations were made on each individual, and the average taken, then we can assume that the intrasubject variability has been averaged out and the variation in the average values is due solely to the intersubject variability. Single observations on individuals clearly contain a mixture of intersubject and intrasubject variation. The *coefficient of variation* (CV%) is the intrasubject standard deviation divided by the mean, expressed as a percentage. It is often quoted as a measure of repeatability for biochemical assays, when an assay is carried out on several occasions on the same sample. It has the advantage of being independent of the units of measurement, but also numerous theoretical disadvantages. It is usually nonsensical to use the coefficient of variation as a measure of between subject variability.

Common questions

When should I use the mean and when should I use the median to describe my data?

It is a commonly held misapprehension that for Normally distributed data one uses the mean, and for non-Normally distributed data one uses the median. Alas this is not so: if the data are Normally distributed the mean and the median will be close; if the data are not Normally distributed then both the mean and the median may give useful information. Consider a variable that takes the value 1 for males and 0 for females. This is clearly not Normally distributed. However, the mean gives the proportion of males in the group, whereas the median merely tells us which group contained more than 50% of the people. Similarly, the mean from ordered categorical variables can be more useful than the median, if the ordered categories can be given meaningful scores. For example, a lecture might be rated as 1 (poor) to 5 (excellent). The usual statistic for summarising the result would be the mean.

In the situation where there is a small group at one extreme of a distribution (for example, annual income) then the median will be more "representative" of the distribution.

My data must have values greater than zero and yet the mean and standard deviation are about the same size. How does this happen?

If data have a very skewed distribution, then the standard deviation will be grossly inflated, and is not a good measure of variability to use. As we have shown, occasionally a transformation of the data, such as a log transform, will render the distribution more symmetrical. Alternatively, quote the interquartile range.

1 Mullee MA. How to choose and use a calculator. In: *How to do it 2*. BMJ Publishing Group, 1995:58–62.

Exercises

Exercise 2.1

In the campaign against smallpox a doctor inquired into the number of times 150 people aged 16 and over in an Ethiopian village had been vaccinated. He obtained the following figures: never, 12 people; once, 24; twice, 42; three times, 38; four times, 30; five times, 4. What is the mean number of times those people had been vaccinated and what is the standard deviation?

Exercise 2.2

Obtain the mean and standard deviation of the data in Exercise 1.1 and an approximate 95% range.

Exercise 2.3

Which points are excluded from the range mean $-2SD$ to mean $+2SD$? What proportion of the data is excluded?

3 Populations and samples

Populations

In statistics the term "population" has a slightly different meaning from the one given to it in ordinary speech. It need not refer only to people or to animate creatures—the population of Britain, for instance or the dog population of London. Statisticians also speak of a population of objects, or events, or procedures, or observations, including such things as the quantity of lead in urine, visits to the doctor, or surgical operations. A population is thus an aggregate of creatures, things, cases and so on.

Although a statistician should clearly define the population he or she is dealing with, they may not be able to enumerate it exactly. For instance, in ordinary usage the population of England denotes the number of people within England's boundaries, perhaps as enumerated at a census. But a physician might embark on a study to try to answer the question "What is the average systolic blood pressure of Englishmen aged 40–59?" But who are the "Englishmen" referred to here? Not all Englishmen live in England, and the social and genetic background of those that do may vary. A surgeon may study the effects of two alternative operations for gastric ulcer. But how old are the patients? What sex are they? How severe is their disease? Where do they live? And so on. The reader needs precise information on such matters to draw valid inferences from the sample that was studied to the population being considered. Statistics such as averages and standard deviations, when taken from populations are referred to as population parameters. They are often denoted by Greek letters: the population mean is denoted by μ (mu) and the standard deviation denoted by σ (lower case sigma).

Samples

A population commonly contains too many individuals to study conveniently, so an investigation is often restricted to one or more samples drawn from it. A well chosen sample will contain most of the information about a particular population parameter but the relation between the sample and the population must be such as to allow true inferences to be made about a population from that sample.

Consequently, the first important attribute of a sample is that every individual in the population from which it is drawn must have a known non-zero chance of being included in it; a natural suggestion is that these chances should be equal. We would like the choices to be made independently; in other words, the choice of one subject will not affect the chance of other subjects being chosen. To ensure this we make the choice by means of a process in which chance alone operates, such as spinning a coin or, more usually, the use of a table of random numbers. A limited table is given in the Appendix (Table F), and more extensive ones have been published.[1-4] A sample so chosen is called a *random sample*. The word "random" does not describe the sample as such but the way in which it is selected.

To draw a satisfactory sample sometimes presents greater problems than to analyse statistically the observations made on it. A full discussion of the topic is beyond the scope of this book, but guidance is readily available.[12] In this book only an introduction is offered.

Before drawing a sample the investigator should define the population from which it is to come. Sometimes he or she can completely enumerate its members before beginning analysis—for example, all the livers studied at necropsy over the previous year, all the patients aged 20–44 admitted to hospital with perforated peptic ulcer in the previous 20 months. In retrospective studies of

23

this kind numbers can be allotted serially from any point in the table to each patient or specimen. Suppose we have a population of size 150, and we wish to take a sample of size five. Table F contains a set of computer generated random digits arranged in groups of five. Choose any row and column, say the last column of five digits. Read only the first three digits, and go down the column starting with the first row. Thus we have 265, 881, 722, etc. If a number appears between 001 and 150 then we include it in our sample. Thus, in order, in the sample will be subjects numbered 24, 59, 107, 73, and 65. If necessary we can carry on down the next column to the left until the full sample is chosen.

The use of random numbers in this way is generally preferable to taking every alternate patient or every fifth specimen, or acting on some other such regular plan. The regularity of the plan can occasionally coincide by chance with some unforeseen regularity in the presentation of the material for study—for example, by hospital appointments being made from patients from certain practices on certain days of the week, or specimens being prepared in batches in accordance with some schedule.

As susceptibility to disease generally varies in relation to age, sex, occupation, family history, exposure to risk, inoculation state, country lived in or visited, and many other genetic or environmental factors, it is advisable to examine samples when drawn to see whether they are, on average, comparable in these respects. The random process of selection is intended to make them so, but sometimes it can by chance lead to disparities. To guard against this possibility the sampling may be *stratified*. This means that a framework is laid down initially, and the patients or objects of the study in a random sample are then allotted to the compartments of the framework. For instance, the framework might have a primary division into males and females and then a secondary division of each of those categories into five age groups, the result being a framework with ten compartments. It is then important to bear in mind that the distributions of the categories on two samples made up on such a framework may be truly comparable, but they will not reflect the distribution of these categories in the population from which the sample is drawn unless the compartments in the framework have been designed with that in mind. For instance, equal numbers might be admitted to the male and female categories, but males and females are not equally numerous in the general

24

population, and their relative proportions vary with age. This is known as *stratified random sampling*. For taking a sample from a long list a compromise between strict theory and practicalities is known as a *systematic random sample*. In this case we choose subjects a fixed interval apart on the list, say every tenth subject, but we choose the starting point within the first interval at random.

Unbiasedness and precision

The terms unbiased and precision have acquired special meanings in statistics. When we say that a measurement is *unbiased* we mean that the average of a large set of unbiased measurements will be close to the true value. When we say it is *precise* we mean that it is repeatable. Repeated measurements will be close to one another, but not necessarily close to the true value. We would like a measurement that is both accurate and precise. Some authors equate unbiasedness with *accuracy*, but this is not universal and others use the term accuracy to mean a measurement that is both unbiased *and* precise. Strike[5] gives a good discussion of the problem.

An estimate of a parameter taken from a random sample is known to be unbiased. As the sample size increases, it gets more precise.

Randomisation

Another use of random number tables is to randomise the allocation of treatments to patients in a clinical trial. This ensures that there is no bias in treatment allocation and, in the long run, the subjects in each treatment group are comparable in both known and unknown prognostic factors. A common method is to use *blocked randomisation*. This is to ensure that at regular intervals there are equal numbers in the two groups. Usual sizes for blocks are two, four, six, eight, and ten. Suppose we chose a block size of ten. A simple method using Table F is to choose the first five unique digits in any row. If we chose the first row, the first five unique digits are 3, 5, 6, 8, and 4. Thus we would allocate the third, fourth, fifth, sixth, and eighth subjects to one treatment and the first, second, seventh, ninth, and tenth to the other. If the block size was less than ten we would ignore digits bigger than the block size. To allocate further subjects to treatment, we carry on

25

along the same row, choosing the next five unique digits for the first treatment. In randomised controlled trials it is advisable to change the block size from time to time to make it more difficult to guess what the next treatment is going to be.

It is important to realise that patients in a randomised trial are *not* a random sample from the population of people with the disease in question but rather a highly selected set of eligible and willing patients. However, randomisation ensures that in the long run any differences in outcome in the two treatment groups are due solely to differences in treatment.

Variation between samples

Even if we ensure that every member of a population has a known, and usually an equal, chance of being included in a sample, it does not follow that a series of samples drawn from one population and fulfilling this criterion will be identical. They will show chance variations from one to another, and the variation may be slight or considerable. For example, a series of samples of the body temperature of healthy people would show very little variation from one to another, but the variation between samples of the systolic blood pressure would be considerable. Thus the variation between samples depends partly on the amount of variation in the population from which they are drawn.

Furthermore, it is a matter of common observation that a small sample is a much less certain guide to the population from which it was drawn than a large sample. In other words, the more members of a population that are included in a sample the more chance will that sample have of accurately representing the population, provided a random process is used to construct the sample. A consequence of this is that, if two or more samples are drawn from a population, the larger they are the more likely they are to resemble each other—again provided that the random technique is followed. Thus the variation between samples depends partly also on the size of the sample. Usually, however, we are not in a position to take a random sample; our sample is simply those subjects available for study. This is a "convenience" sample. For valid generalisations to be made we would like to assert that our sample is in some way representative of the population as a whole and for this reason the

26

first stage in a report is to describe the sample, say by age, sex, and disease status, so that other readers can decide if it is representative of the type of patients they encounter.

Standard error of the mean

If we draw a series of samples and calculate the mean of the observations in each, we have a series of means. These means generally conform to a Normal distribution, and they often do so even if the observations from which they were obtained do not (see Exercise 3.3). This can be proven mathematically and is known as the "Central Limit Theorem". The series of means, like the series of observations in each sample, has a standard deviation. The standard error of the mean of one sample is an estimate of the standard deviation that would be obtained from the means of a large number of samples drawn from that population.

As noted above, if random samples are drawn from a population their means will vary from one to another. The variation depends on the variation of the population and the size of the sample. We do not know the variation in the population so we use the variation in the sample as an estimate of it. This is expressed in the standard deviation. If we now divide the standard deviation by the square root of the number of observations in the sample we have an estimate of the standard error of the mean, $SEM = SD/\sqrt{n}$. It is important to realise that we do not have to take repeated samples in order to estimate the standard error, there is sufficient information within a single sample. However, the conception is that *if* we were to take repeated random samples from the population, this is how we would expect the mean to vary, purely by chance.

A general practitioner in Yorkshire has a practice which includes part of a town with a large printing works and some of the adjacent sheep farming country. With her patients' informed consent she has been investigating whether the diastolic blood pressure of men aged 20–44 differs between the printers and the farm workers. For this purpose she has obtained a random sample of 72 printers and 48 farm workers and calculated the mean and standard deviations, as shown in Table 3.1.

To calculate the standard errors of the two mean blood pressures the standard deviation of each sample is divided by the square root of the number of the observations in the sample.

27

$$\text{Printers: SEM} = 4 \cdot 5 / \sqrt{72} = 0 \cdot 53 \text{ mmHg.}$$

$$\text{Farmers: SEM} = 4 \cdot 2 / \sqrt{48} = 0 \cdot 61 \text{ mmHg.}$$

These standard errors may be used to study the significance of the difference between the two means, as described in successive chapters.

Table 3.1 *Mean diastolic blood pressures of printers and farmers*

	Number	Mean diastolic blood pressure (mmHg)	Standard deviation (mmHg)
Printers	72	88	4·5
Farmers	48	79	4·2

Standard error of a proportion or a percentage

Just as we can calculate a standard error associated with a mean so we can also calculate a standard error associated with a percentage or a proportion. Here the size of the sample will affect the size of the standard error but the amount of variation is determined by the value of the percentage or proportion in the population itself, and so we do not need an estimate of the standard deviation. For example, a senior surgical registrar in a large hospital is investigating acute appendicitis in people aged 65 and over. As a preliminary study he examines the hospital case notes over the previous 10 years and finds that of 120 patients in this age group with a diagnosis confirmed at operation 73 (60·8%) were women and 47 (39·2%) were men.

If p represents one percentage, $100 - p$ represents the other. Then the standard error of each of these percentages is obtained by (1) multiplying them together, (2) dividing the product by the number in the sample, and (3) taking the square root:

$$\text{SE percentage} = \sqrt{\frac{p(100 - p)}{n}}$$

which for the appendicitis data given above is as follows:

$$\text{SE percentage} = \sqrt{\frac{60\cdot8 \times 39\cdot2}{120}} = 4\cdot46$$

Problems with non-random samples

In general we do not have the luxury of a random sample; we have to make do with what is available, a *"convenience sample"*. In order to be able to make generalisations we should investigate whether biases could have crept in, which mean that the patients available are not typical. Common biases are:

- hospital patients are not the same as ones seen in the community;
- volunteers are not typical of non-volunteers;
- patients who return questionnaires are different from those who do not.

In order to persuade the reader that the patients included are typical it is important to give as much detail as possible at the beginning of a report of the selection process and some demographic data such as age, sex, social class and response rate.

Common questions

Given measurements on a sample, what is the difference between a standard deviation and a standard error?

A standard deviation is a sample estimate of the population parameter σ; that is, it is an estimate of the variability of the observations. Since the population is unique, it has a unique standard deviation, which may be large or small depending on how variable the observations are. We would not expect the sample standard deviation to get smaller because the sample gets larger. However, a large sample would provide a more precise estimate of the population standard deviation σ than a small sample.

A standard error, on the other hand, is a measure of precision of an estimate of a population parameter. A standard error is always attached to a parameter, and one can have standard errors of any estimate, such as mean, median, fifth centile, even the standard error

29

of the standard deviation. Since one would expect the precision of the estimate to increase with the sample size, the standard error of an estimate will decrease as the sample size increases.

When should I use a standard deviation to describe data and when should I use a standard error?

It is a common mistake to try and use the standard error to describe data. Usually it is done because the standard error is smaller, and so the study appears more precise. If the purpose is to describe the data (for example so that one can see if the patients are typical) and if the data are plausibly Normal, then one should use the standard deviation (mnemonic D for Description and D for Deviation). If the purpose is to describe the outcome of a study, for example to estimate the prevalence of a disease, or the mean height of a group, then one should use a standard error (or, better, a confidence interval; see Chapter 4) (mnemonic E for Estimate and E for Error).

1 Altman DG. *Practical Statistics for Medical Research*. London: Chapman & Hall, 1991.
2 Armitage P, Berry G. *Statistical Methods in Medical Research*. Oxford: Blackwell Scientific Publications, 1994.
3 Campbell MJ, Machin D. *Medical Statistics: A Commonsense Approach*. 2nd ed. Chichester: John Wiley, 1993.
4 Fisher RA, Yates F. *Statistical Tables for Biological, Agricultural and Medical Research*, 6th ed. London: Longman, 1974.
5 Strike PW. Measurement and control. *Statistical Methods in Laboratory Medicine*. Oxford: Butterworth–Heinemann, 1991:255.

Exercises

Exercise 3.1

The mean urinary lead concentration in 140 children was 2·18 μmol/24 h, with standard deviation 0·87. What is the standard error of the mean?

Exercise 3.2

In Table F, what is the distribution of the digits, and what are the mean and standard deviation?

Exercise 3.3

For the first column of five digits in Table F take the mean value of the five digits and do this for all rows of five digits in the column. What would you expect a histogram of the means to look like? What would you expect the mean and standard deviation to be?

4 Statements of probability and confidence intervals

We have seen that when a set of observations have a Normal distribution multiples of the standard deviation mark certain limits on the scatter of the observations. For instance, 1·96 (or approximately 2) standard deviations above and 1·96 standard deviations below the mean ($\pm 1·96$ SD) mark the points within which 95% of the observations lie.

Reference ranges

We noted in Chapter 1 that 140 children had a mean urinary lead concentration of 2·18 μmol/24 h, with standard deviation 0·87. The points that include 95% of the observations are $2·18 \pm (1·96 \times 0·87)$, giving a range of 0·48 to 3·89. One of the children had a urinary lead concentration of just over 4·0 μmol/ 24 h. This observation is greater than 3·89 and so falls in the 5% beyond the 95% probability limits. We can say that the probability of each of such observations occurring is 5% or less. Another way of looking at this is to see that if one chose one child at random out of the 140, the chance that their urinary lead concentration exceeded 3·89 or was less than 0·48 is 5%. This probability is usually used expressed as a fraction of 1 rather than of 100, and written $P < 0·05$.

Standard deviations thus set limits about which probability statements can be made. Some of these are set out in Table A (Appendix). To use Table A to estimate the probability of finding an observed value, say a urinary lead concentration of 4·8 μmol/24 h, in sampling from the same population of observations as the 140 children provided, we proceed as follows. The distance of the new observation from the mean is 4·8–2·18=2·62. How many standard deviations does this represent? Dividing the difference by the standard deviation gives 2·62/0·87=3·01. This number is greater than 2·576 but less than 3·291 in Table A, so the probability of finding a deviation as large or more extreme than this lies between 0·01 and 0·001, which may be expressed as 0·001<P<0·01. In fact Table A shows that the probability is very close to 0·0027. This probability is small, so the observation probably did not come from the same population as the 140 other children.

To take another example, the mean diastolic blood pressure of printers was found to be 88 mmHg and the standard deviation 4·5 mmHg. One of the printers had a diastolic blood pressure of 100 mmHg. The mean plus or minus 1·96 times its standard deviation gives the following two figures:

$$88 + (1·96 \times 4·5) = 96·8 \, mmHg$$
$$88 - (1·96 \times 4·5) = 79·2 \, mmHg.$$

We can say therefore that only 1 in 20 (or 5%) of printers in the population from which the sample is drawn would be expected to have a diastolic blood pressure below 79 or above about 97 mmHg. These are the 95% limits. The 99·73% limits lie three standard deviations below and three above the mean. The blood pressure of 100 mmHg noted in one printer thus lies beyond the 95% limit of 97 but within the 99·73% limit of 101·5 ($=88 + (3 \times 4·5)$).

The 95% limits are often referred to as a "reference range". For many biological variables, they define what is regarded as the normal (meaning standard or typical) range. Anything outside the range is regarded as abnormal. Given a sample of disease free subjects, an alternative method of defining a normal range would be simply to define points that exclude 2·5% of subjects at the top end and 2·5% of subjects at the lower end. This would give an *empirical normal range*. Thus in the 140 children we might choose

32

to exclude the three highest and three lowest values. However, it is much more efficient to use the mean ± 2 SD, unless the data set is quite large (say >400).

Confidence intervals

The means and their standard errors can be treated in a similar fashion. If a series of samples are drawn and the mean of each calculated, 95% of the means would be expected to fall within the range of two standard errors above and two below the mean of these means. This common mean would be expected to lie very close to the mean of the population. So the standard error of a mean provides a statement of probability about the difference between the mean of the population and the mean of the sample.

In our sample of 72 printers, the standard error of the mean was 0·53 mmHg. The sample mean plus or minus 1·96 times its standard error gives the following two figures:

$$88 + (1·96 \times 0·53) = 89·04 \text{ mmHg}$$
$$88 - (1·96 \times 0·53) = 86·96 \text{ mmHg.}$$

This is called the 95% *confidence interval*, and we can say that there is only a 5% chance that the range 86·96 to 89·04 mmHg excludes the mean of the population. If we take the mean plus or minus three times its standard error, the range would be 86·41 to 89·59. This is the 99·73% confidence interval, and the chance of this range excluding the population mean is 1 in 370. Confidence intervals provide the key to a useful device for arguing from a sample back to the population from which it came.

The standard error for the percentage of male patients with appendicitis, described in Chapter 3, was 4·46. This is also the standard error of the percentage of female patients with appendicitis, since the formula remains the same if p is replaced by $100 - p$. With this standard error we can get 95% confidence intervals on the two percentages:

$$60·8 \pm (1·96 \times 4·46) = 52·1 \text{ and } 69·5$$
$$39·2 \pm (1·96 \times 4·46) = 30·5 \text{ and } 47·9.$$

These confidence intervals exclude 50%. Can we conclude that males are more likely to get appendicitis? This is the subject of the rest of the book, namely *inference*.

With small samples—say under 30 observations—larger multiples of the standard error are needed to set confidence limits. This subject is discussed under the *t* distribution (Chapter 7).

There is much confusion over the interpretation of the probability attached to confidence intervals. To understand it we have to resort to the concept of repeated sampling. Imagine taking repeated samples of the same size from the same population. For each sample calculate a 95% confidence interval. Since the samples are different, so are the confidence intervals. We know that 95% of these intervals will include the population parameter. However, without any additional information we cannot say which ones! Thus with only one sample, and no other information about the population parameter, we can say there is a 95% chance of including the parameter in our interval. Note that this does *not* mean that we would expect with 95% probability that the mean from another sample is in this interval. In this case we are considering differences between two sample means, which is the subject of the next chapter.

Common questions

What is the difference between a reference range and a confidence interval?

There is precisely the same relationship between a reference range and a confidence interval as between the standard deviation and the standard error. The reference range refers to *individuals* and the confidence intervals to *estimates*. It is important to realise that samples are not unique. Different investigators taking samples from the same population will obtain different estimates, and have different 95% confidence intervals. However, we know that for 95 of every 100 investigators the confidence interval will include the population mean interval.

When should one quote a confidence interval?

There is now a great emphasis on confidence intervals in the literature, and some authors attach them to every estimate they make. In general, unless the main purpose of a study is to actually estimate a mean or a percentage, confidence intervals are best

34

restricted to the main outcome of a study, which is usually a *contrast* (that is, a difference) between means or percentages. This is the topic for the next two chapters.

Exercises

Exercise 4.1

A count of malaria parasites in 100 fields with a 2 mm oil immersion lens gave a mean of 35 parasites per field, standard deviation 11·6 (note that, although the counts are quantitative discrete, the counts can be assumed to follow a Normal distribution because the average is large). On counting one more field the pathologist found 52 parasites. Does this number lie outside the 95% reference range? What is the reference range?

Exercise 4.2

What is the 95% confidence interval for the mean of the population from which this sample count of parasites was drawn?

5 Differences between means: type I and type II errors and power

We saw in Chapter 3 that the mean of a sample has a standard error, and a mean that departs by more than twice its standard error from the population mean would be expected by chance only in about 5% of samples. Likewise, the difference between the means of two samples has a standard error. We do not usually know the population mean, so we may suppose that the mean of one of our samples estimates it. The sample mean may happen to be identical with the population mean but it more probably lies somewhere above or below the population mean, and there is a 95% chance that it is within 1·96 standard errors of it.

Consider now the mean of the second sample. If the sample comes from the same population its mean will also have a 95% chance of lying within 1·96 standard errors of the population mean but if we do not know the population mean we have only the means of our samples to guide us. Therefore, if we want to know whether they are likely to have come from the same population, we ask whether they lie within a certain range, represented by their standard errors, of each other.

Large sample standard error of difference between means

If SD_1 represents the standard deviation of sample 1 and SD_2 the standard deviation of sample 2, n_1 the number in sample 1 and n_2 the number in sample 2, the formula denoting the standard error of the difference between two means is:

$$SE\,(diff) = \sqrt{\left(\frac{SD_1^2}{n_1} + \frac{SD_2^2}{n_2}\right)} \tag{5.1}$$

The computation is straightforward.

Square the standard deviation of sample 1 and divide by the number of observations in the sample:

$$SD^2{}_1/n_1 \tag{1}$$

Square the standard deviation of sample 2 and divide by the number of observations in the sample:

$$SD^2{}_2/n_2 \tag{2}$$

Add (1) and (2).

$$\frac{SD_1^2}{n_1} + \frac{SD_2^2}{n_2}$$

Take the square root, to give equation (5.1).

This is the standard error of the difference between the two means.

Large sample confidence interval for the difference in two means

From the data in Table 3.1 the general practitioner wants to compare the mean of the printers' blood pressures with the mean of the farmers' blood pressures. The figures are set out first as in Table 5.1 (which repeats Table 3.1).

37

Table 5.1   *Mean diastolic blood pressures of printers and farmers*

	Number	Mean diastolic blood pressure (mmHg)	Standard deviation
Printers	72	88	4·5
Farmers	48	79	4·2

Analysing these figures in accordance with the formula given above, we have:

$$\text{SE (diff)} = \sqrt{\left(\frac{4\cdot5^2}{72} + \frac{4\cdot2^2}{48}\right)} = 0\cdot81 \text{ mmHg.}$$

The difference between the means is $88 - 79 = 9$ mmHg.

For large samples we can calculate a 95% confidence interval for the difference in means as

$$9 - 1\cdot96 \times 0\cdot81 \text{ to } 9 + 1\cdot96 \times 0\cdot81$$

which is

$$7\cdot41 \text{ to } 10\cdot59 \text{ mmHg.}$$

For a small sample we need to modify this procedure, as described in Chapter 7.

Null hypothesis and type I error

In comparing the mean blood pressures of the printers and the farmers we are testing the hypothesis that the two samples came from the same population of blood pressures. The hypothesis that there is no difference between the population from which the printers' blood pressures were drawn and the population from which the farmers' blood pressures were drawn is called the *null hypothesis*.

But what do we mean by "no difference"? Chance alone will almost certainly ensure that there is some difference between the *sample* means, for they are most unlikely to be identical. Consequently we set limits within which we shall regard the samples as not having any significant difference. If we set the limits at twice the standard error of the difference, and regard a mean outside this range as coming from another population, we shall on average be wrong about one time in 20 if the null hypothesis is in fact true. If we do obtain a mean difference bigger than two standard errors we are faced with two choices: either an unusual event has happened, or the null hypothesis is incorrect. Imagine tossing a coin five times and getting the same face each time. This has nearly the same probability (6·3%) as obtaining a mean difference bigger than two standard errors when the null hypothesis is true. Do we regard it as a lucky event or suspect a biased coin? If we are unwilling to believe in unlucky events, we reject the null hypothesis, in this case that the coin is a fair one.

To reject the null hypothesis when it is true is to make what is known as a *type I error*. The level at which a result is declared significant is known as the type I error rate, often denoted by α. We try to show that a null hypothesis is *unlikely*, not its converse (that it is likely), so a difference which is greater than the limits we have set, and which we therefore regard as "significant", makes the null hypothesis *unlikely*. However, a difference within the limits we have set, and which we therefore regard as "non-significant", does not make the hypothesis likely.

A range of not more than two standard errors is often taken as implying "no difference" but there is nothing to stop investigators choosing a range of three standard errors (or more) if they want to reduce the chances of a type I error.

Testing for differences of two means

To find out whether the difference in blood pressure of printers and farmers could have arisen by chance the general practitioner erects the null hypothesis that there is no significant difference between them. The question is, how many multiples of its standard error does the difference in means difference represent? Since the difference in means is 9 mmHg and its standard error is 0·81 mmHg, the answer is: 9/0·81 = 11·1. We usually denote the ratio of an estimate to its standard error by "z", that is, z = 11·1. Reference to Table A (Appendix) shows that z is far beyond the figure of 3·291 standard deviations, representing a probability of

0·001 (or 1 in 1000). The probability of a difference of 11·1 standard errors or more occurring by chance is therefore exceedingly low, and correspondingly the null hypothesis that these two samples came from the same population of observations is exceedingly unlikely. The probability is known as the *P value* and may be written $P \ll 0.001$.

It is worth recapping this procedure, which is at the heart of statistical inference. Suppose that we have samples from two groups of subjects, and we wish to see if they could plausibly come from the same population. The first approach would be to calculate the difference between two statistics (such as the means of the two groups) and calculate the 95% confidence interval. If the two samples were from the same population we would expect the confidence interval to include zero 95% of the time, and so if the confidence interval excludes zero we suspect that they are from a different population. The other approach is to compute the probability of getting the observed value, or *one that is more extreme*, if the null hypothesis were correct. This is the P value. If this is less than a specified level (usually 5%) then the result is declared significant and the null hypothesis is rejected. These two approaches, the estimation and hypothesis testing approach, are complementary. Imagine if the 95% confidence interval just captured the value zero, what would be the P value? A moment's thought should convince one that it is 2·5%. This is known as a *one sided P value*, because it is the probability of getting the observed result or one bigger than it. However, the 95% confidence interval is two sided, because it excludes not only the 2·5% above the upper limit but also the 2·5% below the lower limit. To support the complementarity of the confidence interval approach and the null hypothesis testing approach, most authorities double the one sided P value to obtain a two sided P value (see below for the distinction between one sided and two sided tests).

Sometimes an investigator knows a mean from a very large number of observations and wants to compare the mean of her sample with it. We may not know the standard deviation of the large number of observations or the standard error of their mean but this need not hinder the comparison if we can assume that the standard error of the mean of the large number of observations is near zero or at least very small in relation to the standard error of the mean of the small sample.

This is because in equation (5.1) for calculating the standard error of the difference between the two means, when n_1 is very large then SD_1^2/n_1 becomes so small as to be negligible. The formula thus reduces to

$$\sqrt{\frac{SD_2^2}{n_2}}$$

which is the same as that for standard error of the sample mean, namely

$$\frac{SD_2}{\sqrt{n_2}}.$$

Consequently we find the standard error of the mean of the sample and divide it into the difference between the means.

For example, a large number of observations has shown that the mean count of erythrocytes in men is $5 \cdot 5 \times 10^{12}/l$. In a sample of 100 men a mean count of $5 \cdot 35$ was found with standard deviation $1 \cdot 1$. The standard error of this mean is $SD/\sqrt{n}$, $1 \cdot 1/\sqrt{100} = 0 \cdot 11$. The difference between the two means is $5 \cdot 5 - 5 \cdot 35 = 0 \cdot 15$. This difference, divided by the standard error, gives $z = 0 \cdot 15/0 \cdot 11 = 1 \cdot 36$. This figure is well below the 5% level of $1 \cdot 96$ and in fact is below the 10% level of $1 \cdot 645$ (see Table A). We therefore conclude that the difference could have arisen by chance.

Alternative hypothesis and type II error

It is important to realise that when we are comparing two groups a non-significant result does not mean that we have proved the two samples come from the same population—it simply means that we have failed to prove that they do *not* come from the population. When planning studies it is useful to think of what differences are likely to arise between the two groups, or what would be clinically worthwhile; for example, what do we expect to be the improved benefit from a new treatment in a clinical trial? This leads to a *study hypothesis*, which is a difference we would like to demonstrate. To contrast the study hypothesis with the null hypothesis, it is often called the *alternative hypothesis*. If we do not

41

reject the null hypothesis when in fact there *is* a difference between the groups we make what is known as a *type II error*. The type II error rate is often denoted as β. The *power* of a study is defined as $1 - \beta$ and is the probability of rejecting the null hypothesis when it is false. The most common reason for type II errors is that the study is too small.

The concept of power is really only relevant when a study is being planned (see Chapter 13 for sample size calculations). After a study has been completed, we wish to make statements not about hypothetical alternative hypotheses but about the data, and the way to do this is with estimates and confidence intervals.[1]

Common questions

Why is the P value not the probability that the null hypothesis is true?

A moment's reflection should convince you that the P value could not be the probability that the null hypothesis is true. Suppose we got exactly the same value for the mean in two samples (if the samples were small and the observations coarsely rounded this would not be uncommon; the difference between the means is zero). The probability of getting the observed result (zero) or a result more extreme (a result that is either positive or negative) is unity, that is we can be certain that we must obtain a result which is positive, negative or zero. However, we can never be certain that the null hypothesis is true, especially with small samples, so clearly the statement that the P value is the probability that the null hypothesis is true is in error. We can think of it as a measure of the strength of evidence against the null hypothesis, but since it is critically dependent on the sample size we should not compare P values to argue that a difference found in one group is more "significant" than a difference found in another.

Exercises

Exercise 5.1

In one group of 62 patients with iron deficiency anaemia the haemoglobin level was 12·2 g/dl, standard deviation 1·8 g/dl; in another group of 35 patients it was 10·9 g/dl, standard deviation 2·1 g/dl.

What is the standard error of the difference between the two means, and what is the significance of the difference? What is the difference? Give an approximate 95% confidence interval for the difference.

Exercise 5.2

If the mean haemoglobin level in the general population is taken as 14·4 g/dl, what is the standard error of the difference between the mean of the first sample and the population mean and what is the significance of this difference?

1 Gardner MJ, Altman DG, editors. *Statistics with Confidence.* London: BMJ Publishing Group, 1989.

6 Differences between percentages and paired alternatives

Standard error of difference between percentages or proportions

The surgical registrar who investigated appendicitis cases, referred to in Chapter 3, wonders whether the percentages of men and women in the sample differ from the percentages of all the other men and women aged 65 and over admitted to the surgical wards during the same period. After excluding his sample of appendicitis cases, so that they are not counted twice, he makes a rough estimate of the number of patients admitted in those 10 years and finds it to be about 12–13 000. He selects a systematic random sample of 640 patients, of whom 363 (56·7%) were women and 277 (43·3%) men.

The percentage of women in the appendicitis sample was 60·8% and differs from the percentage of women in the general surgical sample by $60·8 - 56·7 = 4·1\%$. Is this difference of any significance? In other words, could this have arisen by chance?

There are two ways of calculating the standard error of the difference between two percentages: one is based on the null hypothesis that the two groups come from the same population; the other on the alternative hypothesis that they are different. For Normally distributed variables these two are the same if the standard deviations are assumed to be the same, but in the binomial case

44

the standard deviations depend on the estimates of the proportions, and so if these are different so are the standard deviations. Usually both methods give almost the same result.

Confidence interval for a difference in proportions or percentages

The calculation of the standard error of a difference in proportions $p_1 - p_2$ follows the same logic as the calculation of the standard error of two means; sum the squares of the individual standard errors and then take the square root. It is based on the alternative hypothesis that there is a real difference in proportions (further discussion on this point is given in Common Questions at the end of this chapter).

$$SE (p_1 - p_2) = \sqrt{\left(\frac{p_1 \times (100 - p_1)}{n_1} + \frac{p_2 \times (100 - p_2)}{n_2}\right)}.$$

Note that this is an approximate formula; the exact one would use the population proportions rather than the sample estimates.

With our appendicitis data we have:

$$\sqrt{\left(\frac{60 \cdot 8 \times 39 \cdot 2}{120} + \frac{56 \cdot 7 \times 43 \cdot 3}{640}\right)} = 4 \cdot 87.$$

Thus a 95% confidence interval for the difference in percentages is

$$4 \cdot 1 - 1 \cdot 96 \times 4 \cdot 87 \text{ to } 4 \cdot 1 + 1 \cdot 96 \times 4 \cdot 87$$
$$= -5 \cdot 4 \text{ to } 13 \cdot 6\%.$$

Significance test for a difference in two proportions

For a significance test we have to use a slightly different formula, based on the null hypothesis that both samples have a common population proportion, estimated by p.

45

$$\text{SE (diff \%)} = \sqrt{\left(\frac{p \times (100 - p)}{n_1} + \frac{p \times (100 - p)}{n_2}\right)}.$$

To obtain p we must amalgamate the two samples and calculate the percentage of women in the two combined; $100 - p$ is then the percentage of men in the two combined. The numbers in each sample are n_1 and n_2.

Number of women in the samples: $73 + 363 = 436$

Number of people in the samples: $120 + 640 = 760$

Percentage of women: $(436 \times 100)/760 = 57 \cdot 4$

Percentage of men: $(324 \times 100)/760 = 42 \cdot 6$

Putting these numbers in the formula, we find the standard error of the difference between the percentages is

$$\sqrt{\left(\frac{57 \cdot 4 \times 42 \cdot 6}{120} + \frac{57 \cdot 4 \times 42 \cdot 6}{640}\right)} = 4 \cdot 92.$$

This is very close to the standard error estimated under the alternative hypothesis.

The difference between the percentage of women (and men) in the two samples was $4 \cdot 1\%$. To find the probability attached to this difference we divide it by its standard error: $z = 4 \cdot 1/4 \cdot 92 = 0 \cdot 83$. From Table A (Appendix) we find that P is about $0 \cdot 4$ and so the difference between the percentages in the two samples could have been due to chance alone, as might have been expected from the confidence interval. Note that this test gives results identical to those obtained by the χ^2 test without continuity correction (described in the next chapter).

Standard error of a total

The total number of deaths in a town from a particular disease varies from year to year. If the population of the town or area where they occur is fairly large, say, some thousands, and provided that the deaths are independent of one another, the standard error of the number of deaths from a specified cause is given approximately by its square root, $\sqrt{n}$. Further, the standard error of the difference between two numbers of deaths, n_1 and n_2, can be taken as $\sqrt{(n_1 + n_2)}$.

This can be used to estimate the significance of a difference between two totals by dividing the difference by its standard error:

$$z = \frac{n_1 - n_2}{\sqrt{(n_1 + n_2)}}. \tag{6.1}$$

It is important to note that the deaths must be independently caused; for example, they must not be the result of an epidemic such as influenza. The reports of the deaths must likewise be independent; for example, the criteria for diagnosis must be consistent from year to year and not suddenly change in accordance with a new fashion or test, and the population at risk must be the same size over the period of study.

In spite of its limitations this method has its uses. For instance, in Carlisle the number of deaths from ischaemic heart disease in 1973 was 276. Is this significantly higher than the total for 1972, which was 246? The difference is 30. The standard error of the difference is $\sqrt{(276 + 246)} = 22{\cdot}8$. We then take $z = 30/22{\cdot}8 = 1{\cdot}313$. This is clearly much less than $1{\cdot}96$ times the standard error at the 5% level of probability. Reference to Table A shows that $P = 0{\cdot}2$. The difference could therefore easily be a chance fluctuation.

This method should be regarded as giving no more than approximate but useful guidance, and is unlikely to be valid over a period of more than very few years owing to changes in diagnostic techniques. An extension of it to the study of paired alternatives follows.

Paired alternatives

Sometimes it is possible to record the results of treatment or some sort of test or investigation as one of two alternatives. For instance, two treatments or tests might be carried out on pairs obtained by matching individuals chosen by random sampling, or the pairs might consist of successive treatments of the same individual (see p. 61 for a comparison of pairs by the *t* test). The result might then be recorded as "responded or did not respond",

47

"improved or did not improve", "positive or negative", and so on.
This type of study yields results that can be set out as shown in
Table 6.1.

Table 6.1

Member of pair receiving treatment A	Member of pair receiving treatment B
Responded	Responded (1)
Responded	Did not respond (2)
Did not respond	Responded (3)
Did not respond	Did not respond (4)

The significance of the results can then be simply tested by
McNemar's test in the following way. Ignore rows (1) and (4), and
examine rows (2) and (3). Let the larger number of pairs in either of
rows (2) or (3) be called n_1 and the smaller number of pairs in either
of those two rows be n_2. We may then use formula (6.1) to obtain
the result, z. This is approximately Normally distributed under the
null hypothesis, and its probability can be read from Table A.

However, in practice, the fairly small numbers that form the
subject of this type of investigation make a correction advisable.
We therefore diminish the difference between n_1 and n_2 by using
the following formula:

$$z = \frac{|n_1 - n_2| - 1}{\sqrt{(n_1 + n_2)}}.$$

where the vertical lines mean "take the absolute value".

Again, the result is Normally distributed, and its probability can
be read from Table A. As for the unpaired case, there is a slightly
different formula for the standard error used to calculate the
confidence interval.[1] Suppose N is the total number of pairs, then

$$SE\ (\text{diff}) = \frac{1}{N} \sqrt{\left(n_1 + n_2 - \frac{(n_1 - n_2)^2}{N} \right)}.$$

For example, a registrar in the gastroenterological unit of a large
hospital in an industrial city sees a considerable number of patients
with severe recurrent aphthous ulcer of the mouth. Claims have
been made that a recently introduced preparation stops the

pain of these ulcers and promotes quicker healing than existing preparations.

Over a period of 6 months the registrar selected every patient with this disorder and paired them off as far as possible by reference to age, sex, and frequency of ulceration. Finally she had 108 patients in 54 pairs. To one member of each pair, chosen by the toss of a coin, she gave treatment A, which she and her colleagues in the unit had hitherto regarded as the best; to the other member she gave the new treatment, B. Both forms of treatment are local applications, and they cannot be made to look alike. Consequently to avoid bias in the assessment of the results a colleague recorded the results of treatment without knowing which patient in each pair had which treatment. The results are shown in Table 6.2.

Table 6.2   Results of treating aphthous ulcer in 54 pairs of patents

Member of pair receiving treatment A	Member of pair receiving treatment B	Pairs of patients
Responded	Responded	16
Responded	Did not respond	23
Did not respond	Responded	10
Did not respond	Did not respond	5
Total		54

Here $n_1 = 23$, $n_2 = 10$. Entering these values in formula (6.1) we obtain

$$z = \frac{(23-10)-1}{\sqrt{(23+10)}} = \frac{12}{\sqrt{33}} = 2 \cdot 089.$$

The probability value associated with 2·089 is about 0·04 (Table A). Therefore we may conclude that treatment A gave significantly better results than treatment B. The standard error for the confidence interval is

$$SE\ (diff) = \frac{1}{54} \times \sqrt{\left((23+10) - \frac{(23-10)^2}{54} \right)}$$

$$= \frac{1}{54} \times \sqrt{\left(33 - \frac{169}{54} \right)}$$

$$= 0 \cdot 101$$

49

The observed difference in proportions is

$$23/54 - 10/54 = 0.241$$

The 95% confidence interval for the difference in proportions is

$$0.241 - 1.96 \times 0.101 \text{ to } 0.241 + 1.96 \times 0.101$$
that is, 0·043 to 0·439.

Although this does not include zero, the confidence interval is quite wide, reflecting uncertainty as to the true difference because the sample size is small. An exact method is also available.[1]

Common questions

Why is the standard error used for calculating a confidence interval for the difference in two proportions different from the standard error used for calculating the significance?

For nominal variables the standard deviation is not independent of the mean. If we suppose that a nominal variable simply takes the value 0 or 1, then the mean is simply the proportion of 1s and the standard deviation is directly dependent on the mean, being largest when the mean is 0·5. The null and alternative hypotheses are hypotheses about means, either that they are the same (null) or different (alternative). Thus for nominal variables the standard deviations (and thus the standard errors) will also be different for the null and alternative hypotheses. For a confidence interval, the alternative hypothesis is assumed to be true, whereas for a significance test the null hypothesis is assumed to be true. In general the difference in the values of the two methods of calculating the standard errors is likely to be small, and use of either would lead to the same inferences. The reason this is mentioned here is that there is a close connection between the test of significance described in this chapter and the χ^2 test described in Chapter 8. The difference in the arithmetic for the significance test, and that for calculating the confidence interval, could lead some readers to believe that they are unrelated, whereas in fact they are complementary. The problem does not arise with continuous variables, where the standard deviation is usually assumed independent of the mean, and is also assumed to be the same value under both the null and alternative hypotheses.

It is worth pointing out that the formula for calculating the standard error of an estimate is not necessarily unique: it depends on underlying assumptions, and so different assumptions or study designs will lead to different estimates for standard errors for data sets that might be numerically identical.

1 Gardner MJ, Altman DG, editors. *Statistics with Confidence.* London: BMJ Publishing, 1989:31.

Exercises

Exercise 6.1

In an obstetric hospital 17·8% of 320 women were delivered by forceps in 1975. What is the standard error of this percentage? In another hospital in the same region 21·2% of 185 women were delivered by forceps. What is the standard error of the difference between the percentages at this hospital and the first? What is the difference between these percentages of forceps delivery with a 95% confidence interval and what is its significance?

Exercise 6.2

A dermatologist tested a new topical application for the treatment of psoriasis on 47 patients. He applied it to the lesions on one part of the patient's body and what he considered to be the best traditional remedy to the lesions on another but comparable part of the body, the choice of area being made by the toss of a coin. In three patients both areas of psoriasis responded; in 28 patients the disease responded to the traditional remedy but hardly or not at all to the new one; in 13 it responded to the new one but hardly or not at all to the traditional remedy; and in four cases neither remedy caused an appreciable response. Did either remedy cause a significantly better response than the other?

7 The *t* tests

Previously we have considered how to test the null hypothesis that there is no difference between the mean of a sample and the population mean, and no difference between the means of two samples. We obtained the difference between the means by subtraction, and then divided this difference by the standard error of the difference. If the difference is 1·96 times its standard error, or more, it is likely to occur by chance with a frequency of only 1 in 20, or less.

With small samples, where more chance variation must be allowed for, these ratios are not entirely accurate because the uncertainty in estimating the standard error has been ignored. Some modification of the procedure of dividing the difference by its standard error is needed, and the technique to use is the *t* test. Its foundations were laid by WS Gosset, writing under the pseudonym "Student" so that it is sometimes known as Student's *t* test. The procedure does not differ greatly from the one used for large samples, but is preferable when the number of observations is less than 60, and certainly when they amount to 30 or less.

The application of the *t* distribution to the following four types of problem will now be considered.

1. The calculation of a confidence interval for a sample mean.
2. The mean and standard deviation of a sample are calculated and a value is postulated for the mean of the population. How

52

significantly does the sample mean differ from the postulated population mean?

3. The means and standard deviations of two samples are calculated. Could both samples have been taken from the same population?

4. Paired observations are made on two samples (or in succession on one sample). What is the significance of the difference between the means of the two sets of observations?

In each case the problem is essentially the same—namely, to establish multiples of standard errors to which probabilities can be attached. These multiples are the number of times a difference can be divided by its standard error. We have seen that with large samples 1·96 times the standard error has a probability of 5% or less, and 2·576 times the standard error a probability of 1% or less (Table A). With small samples these multiples are larger, and the smaller the sample the larger they become.

Confidence interval for the mean from a small sample

A rare congenital disease, Everley's syndrome, generally causes a reduction in concentration of blood sodium. This is thought to provide a useful diagnostic sign as well as a clue to the efficacy of treatment. Little is known about the subject, but the director of a dermatological department in a London teaching hospital is known to be interested in the disease and has seen more cases than anyone else. Even so, he has seen only 18. The patients were all aged between 20 and 44.

The mean blood sodium concentration of these 18 cases was 115 mmol/l, with standard deviation of 12 mmol/l. Assuming that blood sodium concentration is Normally distributed what is the 95% confidence interval within which the mean of the total population of such cases may be expected to lie?

The data are set out as follows:

Number of observations	18
Mean blood sodium concentration	115 mmol/l
Standard deviation	12 mmol/l
Standard error of mean	$SD/\sqrt{n} = 12/\sqrt{18} = 2{\cdot}83$ mmol/l

To find the 95% confidence interval above and below the mean we now have to find a multiple of the standard error. In large samples we have seen that the multiple is 1·96 (Chapter 4). For small samples we use the table of *t* given in Table B (Appendix). As the sample becomes smaller *t* becomes larger for any particular level of probability. Conversely, as the sample becomes larger *t* becomes smaller and approaches the values given in Table A, reaching them for infinitely large samples.

Since the size of the sample influences the value of *t*, the size of the sample is taken into account in relating the value of *t* to probabilities in the table. Some useful parts of the full *t* table appear in Table B. The left hand column is headed d.f. for "degrees of freedom". The use of these was noted in the calculation of the standard deviation (Chapter 2). In practice the degrees of freedom amount in these circumstances to one less than the number of observations in the sample. With these data we have $18 - 1 = 17$ d.f. This is because only 17 observations plus the total number of observations are needed to specify the sample, the 18th being determined by subtraction.

To find the number by which we must multiply the standard error to give the 95% confidence interval we enter Table B at 17 in the left hand column and read across to the column headed 0·05 to discover the number 2·110. The 95% confidence intervals of the mean are now set as follows:

$$\text{Mean} + 2 \cdot 110 \text{ SE to Mean} - 2 \cdot 110 \text{ SE}$$

which gives us:

$$115 - (2 \cdot 110 \times 2 \cdot 83) \text{ to } 115 + 2 \cdot 110 \times 2 \cdot 83$$
$$\text{or } 109 \cdot 03 \text{ to } 120 \cdot 97 \text{ mmol/l.}$$

We may then say, with a 95% chance of being correct, that the range 109·03 to 120·97 mmol/l includes the population mean.

Likewise from Table B the 99% confidence interval of the mean is as follows:

$$\text{Mean} + 2 \cdot 898 \text{ SE to Mean} - 2 \cdot 898 \text{ SE}$$

which gives:

$$115 - (2\cdot898 \times 2\cdot83) \text{ to } 115 + (2\cdot898 \times 2\cdot83)$$
$$\text{or } 106\cdot80 \text{ to } 123\cdot20 \text{ mmol/l.}$$

Difference of sample mean from population mean (one sample *t* test)

Estimations of plasma calcium concentration in the 18 patients with Everley's syndrome gave a mean of 3·2 mmol/l, with standard deviation 1·1. Previous experience from a number of investigations and published reports had shown that the mean was commonly close to 2·5 mmol/l in healthy people aged 20–44, the age range of the patients. Is the mean in these patients abnormally high?

We set the figures out as follows:

Mean of general population, μ	2·5 mmol/l
Mean of sample, $\bar{x}$	3·2 mmol/l
Standard deviation of sample, SD	1·1 mmol/l
Standard error of sample mean, SD/$\sqrt{}$ n = 1·1$\sqrt{}$18	0·26 mmol/l
Difference between means $\mu - \bar{x} = 2\cdot5 - 3\cdot2$	−0·7 mmol/l

t = difference between means divided by standard error of sample mean

$$t = \frac{\mu - \bar{x}}{SD/\sqrt{n}} = \frac{-0\cdot7}{0\cdot26} = -2\cdot69$$

Degrees of freedom, $n - 1 = 18 - 1 = 17$.

Ignoring the sign of the *t* value, and entering Table B at 17 degrees of freedom, we find that 2·69 comes between probability values of 0·02 and 0·01, in other words between 2% and 1% and so 0·01<P<0·02. It is therefore unlikely that the sample with mean 3·2 came from the population with mean 2·5, and we may conclude that the sample mean is, at least statistically, unusually high. Whether it should be regarded clinically as abnormally high is something that needs to be considered separately by the physician in charge of that case.

Difference between means of two samples

Here we apply a modified procedure for finding the standard error of the difference between two means and testing the size of the difference by this standard error (see Chapter 5 for large samples). For large samples we used the standard deviation of each sample, computed separately, to calculate the standard error of the difference between the means. For small samples we calculate a combined standard deviation for the two samples.

The assumptions are:

1. that the data are quantitative and plausibly Normal
2. that the two samples come from distributions that may differ in their mean value, but not in the standard deviation
3. that the observations are independent of each other.

The third assumption is the most important. In general, repeated measurements on the same individual are not independent. If we had 20 leg ulcers on 15 patients, then we have only 15 independent observations.

The following example illustrates the procedure.

The addition of bran to the diet has been reported to benefit patients with diverticulosis. Several different bran preparations are available, and a clinician wants to test the efficacy of two of them on patients, since favourable claims have been made for each. Among the consequences of administering bran that requires testing is the transit time through the alimentary canal. Does it differ in the two groups of patients taking these two preparations?

The null hypothesis is that the two groups come from the same population. By random allocation the clinician selects two groups of patients aged 40–64 with diverticulosis of comparable severity. Sample 1 contains 15 patients who are given treatment A, and sample 2 contains 12 patients who are given treatment B. The transit times of food through the gut are measured by a standard technique with marked pellets and the results are recorded, in order of increasing time, in Table 7.1.

These data are shown in Figure 7.1. The assumption of approximate Normality and equality of variance are satisfied. The design suggests that the observations are indeed independent. Since

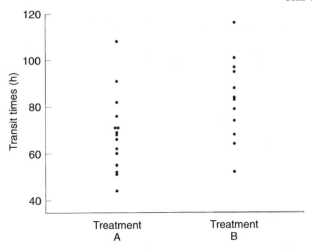

Figure 7.1   Transit times for two bran preparations.

Table 7.1   Transit times of marker pellets through the alimentary canal of patients with diverticulosis on two types of treatment: unpaired comparison

	Transit times (h)	
	Sample 1 (Treatment A)	Sample 2 (Treatment B)
	44	52
	51	64
	52	68
	55	74
	60	79
	62	83
	66	84
	68	88
	69	95
	71	97
	71	101
	76	116
	82	
	91	
	108	
Total	1026	1001
Mean	68·40	83·42

it is possible for the difference in mean transit times for A–B to be positive or negative, we will employ a two sided test.

With treatment A the mean transit time was 68·40 h and with treatment B 83·42 h. What is the significance of the difference, 15·02 h?

The procedure is as follows:

Obtain the standard deviation in sample 1: s_1

Obtain the standard deviation in sample 2: s_2

Multiply the square of the standard deviation of sample 1 by the degrees of freedom, which is the number of subjects minus one:

$$(n_1 - 1)s_1^2$$

Repeat for sample 2

$$(n_2 - 1)s_2^2$$

Add the two together and divide by the total degrees of freedom

$$s_p^2 = \frac{(n_1 - 1)s_1^2 + (n_2 - 1)s_2^2}{n_1 + n_2 - 2}.$$

The standard error of the difference between the means is

$$SE(\bar{x}_1 - \bar{x}_2) = \sqrt{\left(\frac{s_p^2}{n_1} + \frac{s_p^2}{n_2}\right)}$$

which can be written

$$SE(\bar{x}_1 - \bar{x}_2) = s_p \sqrt{\left(\frac{1}{n_1} + \frac{1}{n_2}\right)}.$$

When the difference between the means is divided by this standard error the result is t. Thus,

$$t = \frac{(\bar{x}_1 - \bar{x}_2)}{\sqrt{\left(\dfrac{s_p^2}{n_1} + \dfrac{s_p^2}{n_2}\right)}}.$$

The table of the t distribution (Table B) which gives two sided P values is entered at $(n_1 - 1) + (n_2 - 1)$ degrees of freedom.
For the transit times of Table 7.1,

Treatment A	Treatment B
$n_1 = 15$	$n_2 = 12$
$\bar{x}_1 = 68\cdot40$	$\bar{x}_2 = 83\cdot42$
$s_1 = 16\cdot47$	$s_2 = 17\cdot63$

$$s_p^2 = \frac{14 \times 271\cdot2609 + 11 \times 310\cdot8169}{(15-1)+(12-1)} = 288\cdot67$$

$$SE\ (\bar{x}_1 - \bar{x}_2) = \sqrt{(288\cdot67/15 + 288\cdot67/12)}$$

$$= \sqrt{288\cdot67(1/15 + 1/12)}$$

$$= 6\cdot580$$

$$t = \frac{83\cdot42 - 68\cdot40}{6\cdot580} = 2\cdot282.$$

Table B shows that at 25 degrees of freedom (that is $(15-1)+(12-1)$), $t=2\cdot282$ lies between $2\cdot060$ and $2\cdot485$. Consequently, $0\cdot02 < P < 0\cdot05$.
    This degree of probability is smaller than the conventional level of 5%. The null hypothesis that there is no difference between the means is therefore somewhat unlikely.
    A 95% confidence interval is given by

$$\bar{x}_1 - \bar{x}_2 \pm t(n_1 + n_2 - 2) \times SE.$$

This becomes

$$83 \cdot 42 - 68 \cdot 40 \pm 2 \cdot 06 \times 6 \cdot 582$$
$$15 \cdot 02 - 13 \cdot 56 \text{ to } 15 \cdot 02 + 13 \cdot 56$$
$$\text{or } 1 \cdot 46 \text{ to } 18 \cdot 58 \, h.$$

Unequal standard deviations

If the standard deviations in the two groups are markedly different, for example if the ratio of the larger to the smaller is greater than two, then one of the assumptions of the *t* test (that the two samples come from populations with the same standard deviation) is unlikely to hold. An approximate test, due to Sattherwaite, and described by Armitage and Berry,[1] which allows for unequal standard deviations, is as follows.

Rather than use the pooled estimate of variance, compute

$$\text{SE}\,(\bar{x}_1 - \bar{x}_2) = \sqrt{\left(\frac{s_1^2}{n_1} + \frac{s_2^2}{n_2}\right)}.$$

This is analogous to calculating the standard error of the difference in two proportions under the alternative hypothesis as described in Chapter 6.

We now compute

$$d = \frac{(\bar{x}_1 - \bar{x}_2)}{\text{SE}\,(\bar{x}_1 - \bar{x}_2)}.$$

We then test this using a *t* statistic, in which the degrees of freedom are:

$$df = \frac{(s_1^2/n_1 + s_2^2/n_2)^2}{[(s_1^2/n_1)^2/(n_1 - 1)] + [(s_2^2/n_2)^2/(n_2 - 1)]}.$$

Although this may look very complicated, it can be evaluated very easily on a calculator without having to write down intermediate steps (see below). It can produce a degree of freedom which is not an integer, and so not available in the tables. In this case one should round to the nearest integer. Many statistical packages now carry out this test as the default, and to get the equal variances *t* statistic one has to specifically ask for it. The unequal variance *t* test tends to be less powerful than the usual *t* test if the variances are in fact the same, since it uses fewer assumptions. However, it should not be used indiscriminantly because, if the standard deviations are different, how can we interpret a non-significant difference in means, for example? Often a better strategy is to try a data transformation, such as taking logarithms as described in Chapter 2. Transformations that render distributions closer to Normality often also make the standard deviations similar. If a log transformation is successful use the usual *t* test on the logged data.

Applying this method to the data of Table 7.1, the calculator method (using a Casio fx-350) for calculating the standard error is:

$$16 \cdot 47 \quad \textbf{Inv } \mathbf{x}^2 \div 15 = +17 \cdot 63 \textbf{ Inv } \mathbf{x}^2 \div 12 = \sqrt{(6 \cdot 6321541)}$$

Store this **Min**

Now calculate d

$$83 \cdot 42 - 68 \cdot 40 = \div MR = (2 \cdot 2647242 = d)$$

To calculate the degrees of freedom start with the denominator:

$$16 \cdot 47 \textbf{ Inv } \mathbf{x}^2 \div 15 = \textbf{Inv } \mathbf{x}^2 \div 14 = \textbf{Min } (23 \cdot 359516)$$

$$17 \cdot 63 \textbf{ Inv } \mathbf{x}^2 \div 12 = \textbf{Inv } \mathbf{x}^2 \div 11 = \textbf{M} + \ (60 \cdot 989359)$$

Now calculate the numerator:

$$16 \cdot 47 \textbf{ Inv } \mathbf{x}^2 \div 15 = +17 \cdot 63 \textbf{ Inv } \mathbf{x}^2 \div 12 = \text{Inv } \mathbf{x}^2 \ (1934 \cdot 7214)$$

Divide the numerator by the denominator:

$$\div \textbf{MR} \ (22 \cdot 9371 = \text{d.f.})$$

Thus d.f. = 22·9, or approximately 23. The tabulated values for 2% and 5% from Table B (p134) are 2·069 and 2·500, and so this gives 0·02<P<0·5 as before. This might be expected, because the standard deviations in the original data set are very similar and the sample sizes are close, and so using the unequal variances *t* test gives very similar results to the *t* test which assumes equal variances.

Difference between means of paired samples (paired *t* test)

When the effects of two alternative treatments or experiments are compared, for example in cross over trials, randomised trials in which randomisation is between matched pairs, or matched case control studies (see Chapter 13), it is sometimes possible to make comparisons in pairs. Matching controls for the matched variables, so can lead to a more powerful study.

The test is derived from the single sample *t* test, using the following assumptions.

1. The data are quantitative
2. The distribution of the *differences* (not the original data), is plausibly Normal.
3. The differences are independent of each other.

The first case to consider is when each member of the sample acts as his own control. Whether treatment A or treatment B is given first or second to each member of the sample should be determined by the use of the table of random numbers (Appendix, Table F). In this way any effect of one treatment on the other, even indirectly through the patient's attitude to treatment, for instance, can be minimised. Occasionally it is possible to give both treatments simultaneously, as in the treatment of a skin disease by applying a remedy to the skin on opposite sides of the body.

Let us use as an example the studies of bran in the treatment of diverticulosis discussed earlier. The clinician wonders whether transit time would be shorter if bran is given in the same dosage in three meals during the day (treatment A) or in one meal (treatment B). A random sample of patients with disease of comparable severity and aged 20–44 is chosen and the two treatments administered on two successive occasions, the order of the treatments also being determined from the table of random

Table 7.2   Transit times of marker pellets through the alimentary canal of 12 patients with diverticulosis on two types of treatment: paired comparison

Patient	Transit times (h)		Difference A–B
	Treatment A	Treatment B	
1	63	55	8
2	54	62	−8
3	79	108	−29
4	68	77	−9
5	87	83	4
6	84	78	6
7	92	79	13
8	57	94	−37
9	66	69	−3
10	53	66	−13
11	76	72	4
12	63	77	−14
Total	842	920	−78
Mean	70·17	76·67	−6·5

numbers. The alimentary transit times and the differences for each pair of treatments are set out in Table 7.2.

In calculating *t* on the paired observations we work with the difference, d, between the members of each pair. Our first task is to find the mean of the differences between the observations and then the standard error of the mean, proceeding as follows:

Find the mean of the differences, d̄.

Find the standard deviation of the differences, SD.

Calculate the standard error of the mean SE (d̄) = SD/$\sqrt{n}$.

To calculate *t*, divide the mean of the differences by the standard error of the mean

$$t = \frac{\bar{d}}{SE(\bar{d})}.$$

The table of the *t* distribution is entered at n − 1 degrees of freedom (number of pairs minus 1). For the data from Table 7.2 we have

$$\bar{d} = -6{\cdot}5$$

$$SD = 15{\cdot}1$$

$$SE(\bar{d}) = 4{\cdot}37$$

$$t = -6{\cdot}5/4{\cdot}37 = -1{\cdot}487.$$

Entering Table B at 11 degrees of freedom $(n-1)$ and ignoring the minus sign, we find that this value lies between $0{\cdot}697$ and $1{\cdot}796$. Reading off the probability value, we see that $0{\cdot}1 < P < 0{\cdot}5$. The null hypothesis is that there is no difference between the mean transit times on these two forms of treatment. From our calculations, it is *not* disproved. However, this does not mean that the two treatments are equivalent. To help us decide this we calculate the confidence interval.

A 95% confidence interval for the mean difference is given by

$$\bar{d} \pm t_{n-1}\, SD.$$

In this case t_{11} at $P = 0{\cdot}05$ is $2{\cdot}201$ (Table B) and so the 95% confidence interval is:

$$-6{\cdot}5 - 2{\cdot}201 \times 4{\cdot}37 \text{ to } -6{\cdot}5 + 2{\cdot}201 \times 4{\cdot}37 \text{ h}.$$

$$\text{or } -16{\cdot}1 \text{ to } 3{\cdot}1 \text{ h}.$$

This is quite wide, so we cannot really conclude that the two preparations are equivalent, and should look to a larger study.

The second case of a paired comparison to consider is when two samples are chosen and each member of sample 1 is paired with one member of sample 2, as in a matched case control study. As the aim is to test the difference, if any, between two types of treatment, the choice of members for each pair is designed to make them as alike as possible. The more alike they are, the more apparent will be any differences due to treatment, because they will not be confused with differences in the results caused by disparities between members of the pair. The likeness within the pairs applies to attributes relating to the study in question. For instance, in a test for a drug reducing blood pressure the colour of the patients' eyes would probably be irrelevant, but their resting diastolic blood pressure could well provide a basis for selecting the pairs. Another (perhaps related) basis is the prognosis for the disease in patients: in general, patients with a similar prognosis are best paired. Whatever criteria are chosen, it is essential that the pairs are constructed before the treatment is given, for the pairing must be uninfluenced by knowledge of the effects of treatment.

Further methods

Suppose we had a clinical trial with more than two treatments. It is not valid to compare each treatment with each other treatment using *t* tests because the overall type I error rate α will be bigger than the conventional level set for each individual test. A method of controlling for this to use a *one way analysis of variance.*[2]

Common questions

Should I test my data for Normality before using the t *test?*

It would seem logical that, because the *t* test assumes Normality, one should test for Normality first. The problem is that the test for Normality is dependent on the sample size. With a small sample a non-significant result does not mean that the data come from a Normal distribution. On the other hand, with a large sample, a significant result does not mean that we could not use the *t* test, because the *t* test is *robust* to moderate departures from Normality—that is, the P value obtained can be validly interpreted. There is something illogical about using one significance test conditional on the results of another significance test. In general it is a matter of knowing and looking at the data. One can "eyeball" the data and if the distributions are not extremely skewed, and particularly if (for the two sample *t* test) the numbers of observations are similar in the two groups, then the *t* test will be valid. The main problem is often that outliers will inflate the standard deviations and render the test less sensitive. Also, it is not generally appreciated that if the data originate from a randomised controlled trial, then the process of randomisation will ensure the validity of the *t* test, irrespective of the original distribution of the data.

65

Should I test for equality of the standard deviations before using the usual t *test?*

The same argument prevails here as for the previous question about Normality. The test for equality of variances is dependent on the sample size. A rule of thumb is that if the ratio of the larger to smaller standard deviation is greater than two, then the unequal variance test should be used. With a computer one can easily do both the equal and unequal variance *t* test and see if the answers differ.

Why should I use a paired test if my data are paired? What happens if I don't?

Pairing provides information about an experiment, and the more information that can be provided in the analysis the more sensitive the test. One of the major sources of variability is between subjects variability. By repeating measures within subjects, each subject acts as its own control, and the between subjects variability is removed. In general this means that if there is a true difference between the pairs the paired test is more likely to pick it up: it is more powerful. When the pairs are generated by matching the matching criteria may not be important. In this case, the paired and unpaired tests should give similar results.

1 Armitage P, Berry G. *Statistical Methods in Medical Research.* 3rd ed. Oxford: Blackwell Scientific Publications, 1994:112–13.
2 Armitage P, Berry G. *Statistical Methods in Medical Research.* 3rd ed. Oxford: Blackwell Scientific Publications, 1994:207–14.

Exercises

Exercise 7.1

In 22 patients with an unusual liver disease the plasma alkaline phosphatase was found by a certain laboratory to have a mean value of 39 King–Armstrong units, standard deviation 3·4 units. What is the 95% confidence interval within which the mean of the population of such cases whose specimens come to the same laboratory may be expected to lie?

Exercise 7.2

In the 18 patients with Everley's syndrome the mean level of plasma phosphate was 1·7 mmol/l, standard deviation 0·8. If the mean level in the general population is taken as 1·2 mmol/l, what is the significance of the difference between that mean and the mean of these 18 patients?

Exercise 7.3

In two wards for elderly women in a geriatric hospital the following levels of haemoglobin were found:

Ward A: 12·2, 11·1, 14·0, 11·3, 10·8, 12·5, 12·2, 11·9, 13·6, 12·7, 13·4, 13·7 g/dl;

Ward B: 11·9, 10·7, 12·3, 13·9, 11·1, 11·2, 13·3, 11·4, 12·0, 11·1 g/dl.

What is the difference between the mean levels in the two wards, and what is its significance? What is the 95% confidence interval for the difference in treatments?

Exercise 7.4

A new treatment for varicose ulcer is compared with a standard treatment on ten matched pairs of patients, where treatment between pairs is decided using random numbers. The outcome is the number of days from start of treatment to healing of ulcer. One doctor is responsible for treatment and a second doctor assesses healing without knowing which treatment each patient had. The following treatment times were recorded.

Standard treatment: 35, 104, 27, 53, 72, 64, 97, 121, 86, 41 days;

New treatment: 27, 52, 46, 33, 37, 82, 51, 92, 68, 62 days.

What are the mean difference in the healing time, the value of *t*, the number of degrees of freedom, and the probability? What is the 95% confidence interval for the difference?

8 The χ^2 tests

The distribution of a categorical variable in a sample often needs to be compared with the distribution of a categorical variable in another sample. For example, over a period of 2 years a psychiatrist has classified by socioeconomic class the women aged 20–64 admitted to her unit suffering from self poisoning—sample A. At the same time she has likewise classified the women of similar age admitted to a gastroenterological unit in the same hospital—sample B. She has employed the Registrar General's five socioeconomic classes, and generally classified the women by reference to their father's or husband's occupation. The results are set out in Table 8.1.

Table 8.1 Distribution by socioeconomic class of patients admitted to self poisoning (sample A) and gastroenterological (sample B) units

Socioeconomic class	Samples		Total	Proportion in group A
	A	B		
	a	b	$n = a+b$	$p = a/n$
I	17	5	22	0·77
II	25	21	46	0·54
III	39	34	73	0·53
IV	42	49	91	0·46
V	32	25	57	0·56
Total	155	134	289	

The psychiatrist wants to investigate whether the distribution of the patients by social class differed in these two units. She therefore erects the null hypothesis that there is no difference between the two distributions. This is what is tested by the chi squared (χ^2) test (pronounced with a hard ch as in "sky"). By default, all χ^2 tests are two sided.

It is important to emphasise here that χ^2 tests may be carried out for this purpose only on the *actual numbers* of occurrences, *not* on percentages, proportions, means of observations, or other derived statistics. Note, we distinguish here the Greek (χ^2) for the test and the distribution and the Roman (X^2) for the calculated statistic, which is what is obtained from the test.

The χ^2 test is carried out in the following steps:

For each observed number (O) in the table find an "expected" number (E); this procedure is discussed below.

Subtract each expected number from each observed number $\quad\quad O - E$

Square the difference $\quad\quad (O - E)^2$

Divide the squares so obtained for each cell of the table by the expected number for that cell $\quad\quad (O - E)^2/E$

X^2 is the sum of $(O - E)^2/E$.

To calculate the expected number for each cell of the table consider the null hypothesis, which in this case is that the numbers in each cell are proportionately the same in sample A as they are in sample B. We therefore construct a parallel table in which the proportions are exactly the same for both samples. This has been done in columns (2) and (3) of Table 8.2. The proportions are obtained from the totals column in Table 8.1 and are applied to the totals row. For instance, in Table 8.2, column (2), $11 \cdot 80 = (22/289) \times 155$; $24 \cdot 67 = (46/289) \times 155$; in column (3) $10 \cdot 20 = (22/289) \times 134$; $21 \cdot 33 = (46/289) \times 134$ and so on.

Thus by simple proportions from the totals we find an expected number to match each observed number. The sum of the expected numbers for each sample must equal the sum of the observed numbers for each sample, which is a useful check. We now subtract each expected number from its corresponding observed number.

Table 8.2   Calculation of the χ^2 test on figures in Table 8.1

	Expected numbers		O − E		$(O-E)^2/E$	
Class	A	B	A	B	A	B
(I)	(2)	(3)	(4)	(5)	(6)	(7)
I	11·80	10·20	5·20	−5·20	2·292	2·651
II	24·67	21·33	0·33	−0·33	0·004	0·005
III	39·15	33·85	−0·15	0·15	0·001	0·001
IV	48·81	42·19	−6·81	6·81	0·950	1·009
V	30·57	26·43	1·43	−1·43	0·067	0·077
Total	155·00	134·00	0	0	3·314	3·833

$X^2 = 3·314 + 3·833 = 7·147$. d.f. = 4. $0·10 < P < 0·50$.

The results are given in columns (4) and (5) of Table 8.2. Here two points may be noted.

1. The sum of these differences always equals zero in each column.
2. Each difference for sample A is matched by the same figure, but with opposite sign, for sample B.

Again these are useful checks.

The figures in columns (4) and (5) are then each squared and divided by the corresponding expected numbers in columns (2) and (3). The results are given in columns (6) and (7). Finally these results, $(O-E)^2/E$, are added. The sum of them is X^2.

A helpful technical procedure in calculating the expected numbers may be noted here. Most electronic calculators allow successive multiplication by a constant multiplier by a short cut of some kind. To calculate the expected numbers a constant multiplier for each sample is obtained by dividing the total of the sample by the grand total for both samples. In Table 8.1 for sample A this is $155/289 = 0·5363$. This fraction is then successively multiplied by 22, 46, 73, 91, and 57. For sample B the fraction is $134/289 = 0·4636$. This too is successively multiplied by 22, 46, 73, 91, and 57.

The results are shown in Table 8.2, columns (2) and (3).

Having obtained a value for $X^2 = \Sigma[(O-E)^2/E]$ we look up in a table of χ^2 distribution the probability attached to it (Appendix, Table C). Just as with the t table, we must enter this table at a certain number of degrees of freedom. To ascertain these requires some care.

When a comparison is made between one sample and another, as in Table 8.1, a simple rule is that the degrees of freedom equal (number of columns minus one) × (number of rows minus one) (not counting the row and column containing the totals). For the data in Table 8.1 this gives $(2-1) \times (5-1) = 4$. Another way of looking at this is to ask for the minimum number of figures that must be supplied in Table 8.1, *in addition* to all the totals, to allow us to complete the whole table. Four numbers disposed anyhow in samples A and B provided they are in separate rows will suffice.

Entering Table C at four degrees of freedom and reading along the row we find that the value of X^2 (7·147) lies between 3·357 and 7·779. The corresponding probability is: $0·10<P<0·50$. This is well above the conventionally significant level of 0·05, or 5%, so the null hypothesis is *not* disproved. It is therefore quite conceivable that in the distribution of the patients between socioeconomic classes the population from which sample A was drawn were the same as the population from which sample B was drawn.

Quick method

The above method of calculating X^2 illustrates the nature of the statistic clearly and is often used in practice. A quicker method, similar to the quick method for calculating the standard deviation, is particularly suitable for use with electronic calculators.[1]

The data are set out as in Table 8.1. Take the left hand column of figures (Sample A) and call each observation a. Their total, which is 155, is then Σa.

Let p = the proportion formed when each observation a is divided by the corresponding figure in the total column. Thus here p in turn equals 17/22, 25/46 ... 32/57.

Let $\bar{p}$ = the proportion formed when the total of the observations in the left hand column, Σa, is divided by the total of all the observations.

Here $\bar{p} = 155/289$. Let $\bar{q} = 1 - \bar{p}$, which is the same as 134/289. Then

$$X^2 = \frac{\Sigma pa - \bar{p}\Sigma a}{\bar{p}\bar{q}}.$$

Calculator procedure

Working with the figures in Table 8.1, we use this formula on an electronic calculator (Casio fx-350) in the following way:

17 **Inv x²** ÷ 22 **Min**

25 **Inv x²** ÷ 46 **M +**

39 **Inv x²** ÷ 73 **M +**

42 **Inv x²** ÷ 91 **M +**

32 **Inv x²** ÷ 57 **M +**

155 **Inv x²** ÷ 289 **M +**

Withdraw result from memory on to display screen

$$\textbf{MR} \ (1 \cdot 7769764)$$

We now have to divide this by $\bar{p} \times \bar{q}$. Here $\bar{p} = 155/289$ and $\bar{q} = 134/289$.

$$1 \cdot 776975 \times (289/155) \times (289/134)$$
$$(\times 289 \div 155 \times 289 \div 134)$$

This gives us $X^2 = 7 \cdot 146$.

The calculation naturally gives the same result if the figures for sample B are used instead of those for sample A. Owing to rounding off of the numbers the two methods for calculating X^2 may lead to trivially different results.

Fourfold tables

A special form of the χ^2 test is particularly common in practice and quick to calculate. It is applicable when the results of an investigation can be set out in a "fourfold table" or "2 × 2 contingency table".

For example, the practitioner whose data we displayed in Table 3.1 believed that the wives of the printers and farmers should be encouraged to breast feed their babies. She has records for her practice going back over 10 years, in which she has noted whether the mother breast fed the baby for at least 3 months or not, and these records show whether the husband was a printer or a sheep farmer (or some other occupation less well represented in her practice). The figures from her records are set out in Table 8.3.

The disparity seems considerable, for, although 28% of the printers' wives breast fed their babies for three months or more, as many as 45% of the farmers' wives did so. What is its significance?

Table 8.3 *Numbers of wives of printers and farmers who breast fed their babies for less than 3 months or for 3 months or more*

	Breast fed for		
	Up to 3 months	3 months or more	Total
Printers' wives	36	14	50
Farmers' wives	30	25	55
Total	66	39	105

The null hypothesis is set up that there is no difference between printers' wives and farmers' wives in the period for which they breast fed their babies. The χ^2 test on a fourfold table may be carried out by a formula that provides a short cut to the conclusion. If a, b, c, and d are the numbers in the cells of the fourfold table as shown in Table 8.4 (in this case Variable 1 is breast feeding (<3 months 0, $\geq$3 months 1) and Variable 2 is husband's occupation (Printer (0) or Farmer (1)), X^2 is calculated from the following formula:

$$X^2 = \frac{(ad-bc)^2(a+b+c+d)}{(a+b)\,(c+d)\,(b+d)\,(a+c)}$$

With a fourfold table there is one degree of freedom in accordance with the rule given earlier.

Table 8.4 *Notation for two group χ^2 test*

		Variable 1		
		0	1	Total
Variable 2	0	a	b	a+b
	1	c	d	c+d
Total		a+c	b+d	a+b+c+d

As many electronic calculators have a capacity limited to eight digits, it is advisable not to do all the multiplication or all the division in one series of operations, lest the number become too big for the display.

Calculator procedure

Multiply a by d and store in memory

Multiply b by c and subtract from memory

Extract difference from memory to display	$ad - bc$
Square the difference	$(ad - bc)^2$
Divide by $a + b$	$\dfrac{(ad - bc)^2}{(a + b)}$
Divide by $c + d$	$\dfrac{(ad - bc)^2}{(a + b)(c + d)}$
Multiply by $a + b + c + d$	$\dfrac{(ad - bc)^2(a + b + c + d)}{(a + b)(c + d)}$
Divide by $b + d$	$\dfrac{(ad - bc)^2(a + b + c + d)}{(a + b)(c + d)(b + d)}$
Divide by $a + c$	$\dfrac{(ad - bc)^2(a + b + c + d)}{(a + b)(c + d)(b + d)(a + c)}$

From Table 8.3 we have

$$\frac{[(36 \times 25) - (30 \times 14)]^2 \times 105}{66 \times 39 \times 55 \times 50} = 3 \cdot 418.$$

Entering the χ^2 table with one degree of freedom we read along the row and find that $3 \cdot 418$ lies between $2 \cdot 706$ and $3 \cdot 841$. Therefore $0 \cdot 05 < P < 0 \cdot 1$. So, despite an apparently considerable difference between the proportions of printers' wives and the farmers' wives breast feeding their babies for 3 months or more, the probability of this result or one more extreme occurring by chance is more than 5%.

We now calculate a confidence interval of the differences between the two proportions, as described in Chapter 6. In this case we use the standard error based on the observed data, not the null hypothesis. We could calculate the confidence interval on either the rows or the columns and it is important that we compare proportions of the outcome variable, that is, breast feeding.

$$P_1 = 14/50 = 0 \cdot 28, \ P_2 = 25/55 = 0 \cdot 45, \ P_1 - P_2 = 0 \cdot 17.$$

$$SE(P_1 - P_2) = \sqrt{\left(\frac{0 \cdot 28 \times 0 \cdot 72}{50} + \frac{0 \cdot 45 \times 0 \cdot 55}{55} \right)} = 0 \cdot 0924.$$

The 95% confidence interval is

$$0 \cdot 17 - 1 \cdot 96 \times 0 \cdot 0924 \ \text{to} \ 0 \cdot 17 + 1 \cdot 96 \times 0 \cdot 0924$$
$$= -0 \cdot 011 \ \text{to} \ 0 \cdot 351$$

Thus the 95% confidence interval is wide, and includes zero, as one might expect because the χ^2 test was not significant at the 5% level.

Increasing the precision of the P value in 2×2 tables

It can be shown mathematically that if X is a Normally distributed variable, mean zero and variance 1, then X^2 has a χ^2 distribution with one degree of freedom. The converse also holds true and we can use this fact to improve the precision of our P values. In the above example we have $X^2 = 3 \cdot 418$, with one degree of freedom. Thus $X = 1 \cdot 85$, and from Table A we find P to be about $0 \cdot 065$. However, we do need the χ^2 tables for more than one degree of freedom.

Small numbers

When the numbers in a 2×2 contingency table are small, the χ^2 approximation becomes poor. The following recommendations may be regarded as a sound guide.[2] In fourfold tables a χ^2 test is inappropriate if the total of the table is less than 20, or if the total lies between 20 and 40 and the smallest expected (not observed) value is less than 5; in contingency tables with more than one degree of freedom it is inappropriate if more than about one fifth of the cells have expected values less than 5 or any cell an expected value of less than 1. An alternative to the χ^2 test for fourfold tables is known as Fisher's Exact test and is described in Chapter 9.

When the values in a fourfold table are fairly small a "correction for continuity" known as the "Yates' correction" may be applied.[3] Although there is no precise rule defining the circumstances in which to use Yates' correction, a common practice is to incorporate it into χ^2 calculations on tables with a total of under 100 or with any cell containing a value less than 10. The χ^2 test on a fourfold table is then modified as follows:

$$\frac{[(\mid ad-bc \mid)-0\cdot5(a+b+c+d)]^2(a+b+c+d)}{(a+b)\,(c+d)\,(b+d)\,(a+c)}$$

The vertical bars on either side of $ad-bc$ mean that the smaller of those two products is taken from the larger. Half the total of the four values is then subtracted from that the difference to provide Yates' correction. The effect of the correction is to reduce the value of X^2.

Applying it to the figures in Table 8.3 gives the following result:

$$\frac{[(36 \times 25)-(30 \times 14)-(105/2)]^2 \times 105}{(66 \times 39 \times 55 \times 50)}=2\cdot711.$$

In this case $X^2=2\cdot711$ falls within the same range of P values as the $X^2=3\cdot418$ we got without Yates' correction $(0\cdot05<P<0\cdot1)$, but the P value is closer to $0\cdot1$ than it was in the previous calculation. In fourfold tables containing lower frequencies than Table 8.3 the reduction in P value by Yates' correction may change a result from significant to non-significant; in any case care should be exercised when making decisions from small samples.

Comparing proportions

Earlier in this chapter we compared two samples by the χ^2 test to answer the question "Are the distributions of the members of these two samples between five classes significantly different?" Another way of putting this is to ask "Are the relative proportions of the two samples the same in each class?"

For example, an industrial medical officer of a large factory wants to immunise the employees against influenza. Five vaccines of various types based on the current viruses are available, but nobody knows which is preferable. From the work force 1350 employees agree to be immunised with one of the vaccines in the first week of December, so the medical officer divides the total into five approximately equal groups. Disparities occur between their total numbers owing to the layout of the factory complex. In the first week of the following March he examines the records he has been keeping to see how many employees got influenza and how many did not. These records are classified by the type of vaccine used (Table 8.5).

Table 8.5 People who did or did not get influenza after inoculation with one of five vaccines

Type of vaccine	Numbers of employees			
	Got influenza	Avoided influenza	Total	Proportion got influenza
I	43	237	280	0·18
II	52	198	250	0·21
III	25	245	270	0·09
IV	48	212	260	0·18
V	57	233	290	0·20
Total	225	1125	1350	

In Table 8.6 the figures are analysed by the χ^2 test. For this we have to determine the expected values. The null hypothesis is that there is no difference between vaccines in their efficacy against influenza. We therefore assume that the proportion of employees contracting influenza is the same for each vaccine as it is for all combined. This proportion is derived from the total who got influenza, and is 225/1350. To find the expected number in each vaccine group who would contract the disease we multiply the actual numbers in the Total column of Table 8.5 by this proportion. Thus $280 \times (225/1350) = 46·7$; $250 \times (225/1350) = 41·7$; and so on. Likewise the proportion who did not get influenza is 1125/1350.

The expected numbers of those who would avoid the disease are calculated in the same way from the totals in Table 8.5, so that $280 \times (1125/1350) = 233\cdot3$; $250 \times (1250/1350) = 208\cdot3$; and so on. The procedure is thus the same as shown in Tables 8.1 and 8.2.

The calculations made in Table 8.6 show that X^2 with four degrees of freedom is $16\cdot564$, and $0\cdot001 < P < 0\cdot01$. This is a highly significant result. But what does it mean?

Table 8.6   *Calculation of χ^2 test on figures in Table 8.5*

Type of vaccine	Expected numbers		O − E		(O − E)²/E	
	Got influenza	Avoided influenza	Got influenza	Avoided influenza	Got influenza	Avoided influenza
I	46·7	233·3	−3·7	3·7	0·293	0·059
II	41·7	208·3	10·3	−10·3	2·544	0·509
III	45·0	225·0	−20·0	20·0	8·889	1·778
IV	43·3	216·7	4·7	−4·7	0·510	0·102
V	48·3	241·7	8·7	−8·7	1·567	0·313
Total	225·0	1125·0	0	0	13·803	2·761

$X^2 = 16\cdot564$, d.f. $= 4$, $0\cdot001 < P < 0\cdot01$.

Splitting of χ^2

Inspection of Table 8.6 shows that the largest contribution to the total X^2 comes from the figures for vaccine III. They are $8\cdot889$ and $1\cdot778$, which together equal $10\cdot667$. If this figure is subtracted from the total X^2, $16\cdot564 - 10\cdot667 = 5\cdot897$. This gives an approximate figure for X^2 for the remainder of the table with three degrees of freedom (by removing the vaccine III we have reduced the table to four rows and two columns). We then find that $0\cdot1 < P < 0\cdot5$, a non-significant result. However, this is only a rough approximation. To check it exactly we apply the X^2 test to the figures in Table 8.4 minus the row for vaccine III. In other words, the test is now performed on the figures for vaccines I, II, IV, and V. On these figures $X^2 = 2\cdot983$; d.f. $= 3$; $0\cdot1 < P < 0\cdot5$. Thus the probability falls within the same broad limits as obtained by the approximate short cut given above. We can conclude that the figures for vaccine III are responsible for the highly significant result of the total X^2 of $16\cdot564$.

78

But this is not quite the end of the story. Before concluding from these figures that vaccine III is superior to the others we ought to carry out a check on other possible explanations for the disparity. The process of randomisation in the choice of the persons to receive each of the vaccines should have balanced out any differences between the groups, but some may have remained by chance. The sort of questions worth examining now are: Were the people receiving vaccine III as likely to be exposed to infection as those receiving the other vaccines? Could they have had a higher level of immunity from previous infection? Were they of comparable socioeconomic status? Of similar age on average? Were the sexes comparably distributed? Although some of these characteristics could have been more or less balanced by stratified randomisation, it is as well to check that they have in fact been equalised before attributing the numeral discrepancy in the result to the potency of the vaccine.

χ^2 Test for trend

Table 8.1 is a 5×2 table, because there are five socioeconomic classes and two samples. Socioeconomic groupings may be thought of as an example of an ordered categorical variable, as there are some outcomes (for example, mortality) in which it is sensible to state that (say) social class II is between social class I and social class III. The χ^2 test described at that stage did not make use of this information; if we had interchanged any of the rows the value of X^2 would have been exactly the same. Looking at the proportions p in Table 8.1 we can see that there is no real ordering by social class in the proportions of self poisoning; social class V is between social classes I and II. However in many cases, when the outcome

Table 8.7 Change in eating poultry in randomised trial[4]

	Intervention	Control	Total	Proportion in intervention	Score
	a	b	n	p = a/n	x
Increase	100	78	178	0·56	1
No change	175	173	348	0·50	0
Decrease	42	59	101	0·42	−1
Total	317	310	627	0·51	

variable is an ordered categorical variable, a more powerful test can be devised which uses this information.

Consider a randomised controlled trial of health promotion in general practice to change people's eating habits.[4] Table 8.7 gives the results from a review at 2 years, to look at the change in the proportion eating poultry.

If we give each category a score x the χ^2 test for trend is calculated in the following way:

$$E_{xp} = \frac{\Sigma ax - \Sigma a \Sigma nx}{N}$$

and

$$E_{xx} = \frac{\Sigma nx^2 - (\Sigma nx)^2}{N}$$

then

$$X^2 = E_{xp}^2 / (E_{xx}\bar{p}\bar{q})$$

where:

N is the total sample size

$\bar{p} = \Sigma a/n$ and $\bar{q} = \Sigma b/N$

$\Sigma a = 317$

$N = 627$

$\Sigma ax = 100 \times 1 + 175 \times 0 - 42 \times 1 = 658$

$\Sigma nx = 178 \times 1 + 348 \times 0 - 101 = 77$

$E_{xp} = 58 - 317 \times 77/627 = 19 \cdot 07$

$\Sigma nx^2 = 178 \times 1^2 + 348 \times 0^2 + 101 \times (-1)^2 = 279$

$(\Sigma nx)^2/N = 77^2/627 = 9 \cdot 46$

Thus

$$E_{xx} = 279 - 9 \cdot 46 = 269 \cdot 54$$

$$\bar{p} = 317/627 = 0 \cdot 5056 \quad \bar{q} = 310/627 = 0 \cdot 4944$$

$$X^2 = 19 \cdot 07^2 / (279 \cdot 54 \times 0 \cdot 5056 \times 0 \cdot 4944) = 5 \cdot 20.$$

This has one degree of freedom because the linear scoring means that when one expected value is given all the others are fixed, and we find p = 0·02. The usual χ^2 test gives a value of $X^2 = 5·51$; d.f. = 2; 0·05<P<0·10. Thus the more sensitive χ^2 test for trend yields a significant result because the test used more information about the experimental design. The values for the scores are to some extent arbitrary. However, it is usual to choose them equally spaced on either side of zero. Thus if there are four groups the scores would be −3, −1, +1, +3, and for five groups −2, −1, 0, +1, +2. The X^2 statistic is quite robust to other values for the scores provided that they are steadily increasing or steadily decreasing.

Note that this is another way of splitting the overall X^2 statistic. The overall X^2 will always be greater than the X^2 for trend, but because the latter uses only one degree of freedom, it is often associated with a smaller probability. Although one is often counselled not to decide on a statistical test after having looked at the data, it is obviously sensible to look at the proportions to see if they are plausibly monotonic (go steadily up or down) with the ordered variable, especially if the overall χ^2 test is non-significant.

Comparison of an observed and a theoretical distribution

In the cases so far discussed the observed values in one sample have been compared with the observed values in another. But sometimes we want to compare the observed values in one sample with a theoretical distribution.

For example, a geneticist has a breeding population of mice in his laboratory. Some are entirely white, some have a small patch of brown hairs on the skin, and others have a large patch. According to the genetic theory for the inheritance of these coloured patches of hair the population of mice should include 51·0% entirely white, 40·8% with a small brown patch, and 8·2% with a large brown patch. In fact, among the 784 mice in the laboratory 380 are entirely white, 330 have a small brown patch, and 74 have a large brown patch. Do the proportions differ from those expected?

81

Table 8.8   Calculation of X^2 for comparison between actual distribution and theoretical distribution

Mice	Observed cases	Theoretical proportions	Expected cases	O−E	(O−E)²/E
Entirely white	380	0·510	400	−20	1·0000
Small brown patch	330	0·408	320	10	0·3125
Large brown patch	74	0·082	64	10	1·5625
Total	784	1·000	784	0	2·8750

The data are set out in Table 8.8. The expected numbers are calculated by applying the theoretical proportions to the total, namely $0·510 \times 784$, $0·408 \times 784$, and $0·082 \times 784$. The degrees of freedom are calculated from the fact that the only constraint is that the total for the expected cases must equal the total for the observed cases, and so the degrees of freedom are the number of rows minus one. Thereafter the procedure is the same as in previous calculations of X^2. In this case it comes to 2·875. The X^2 table is entered at two degrees of freedom. We find that $0·2 < P < 0·3$. Consequently the null hypothesis of no difference between the observed distribution and the theoretically expected one is *not* disproved. The data conform to the theory.

McNemar's test

McNemar's test for paired nominal data was described in Chapter 6, using a Normal approximation. In view of the relationship between the Normal distribution and the χ^2 distribution with one degree of freedom, we can recast the McNemar test as a variant of a χ^2 test. The results are often expressed as in Table 8.9.

Table 8.9   Notation for the McNemar test

		First subject of pair		
		Variable 1		
	Variable 2	0	1	Total
2nd subject	0	e	f	e+f
of pair	1	g	h	g+h
Total		e+g	f+h	n

Table 8.10 Data from Table 6.1 for McNemar's test

		First subject of pair	
		Responded	Did not respond
2nd subject	Responded	16	10
of pair	Did not respond	23	5

McNemar's test is then

$$X^2 = \frac{(f-g)^2}{(f+g)} \text{ with 1 d.f.,}$$

or with a continuity correction

$$X_c^2 = \frac{(|f-g|-1)^2}{(f+g)} \text{ with 1 d.f.}$$

The data from Table 6.1 are recast as shown in Table 8.10. Thus

$$X^2 = \frac{(10-23)^2}{(10+23)} = 5.12,$$

or

$$X_c^2 = \frac{(|10-23|-1)^2}{(10+23)} = 4.36.$$

From Table C (Appendix) we find that for both χ^2 values $0.02 < P < 0.05$. The result is identical to that given using the Normal approximation described in Chapter 6, which is the square root of this result.

Extensions of the χ^2 test

If the outcome variable in a study is nominal, the χ^2 test can be extended to look at the effect of more than one input variable, for example to allow for confounding variables. This is most easily done using *multiple logistic regression*, a generalisation of *multiple*

83

regression, which is described in Chapter 11. If the data are matched, then a further technique (*conditional logistic regression*) should be employed. This is described in advanced textbooks and will not be discussed further here.

Common questions

I have matched data, but the matching criteria were very weak. Should I use McNemar's test?

The general principle is that if the data are matched in any way, the analysis should take account of it. If the matching is weak then the matched analysis and the unmatched analysis should agree. In some cases when there are a large number of pairs with the same outcome, it would appear that the McNemar's test is discarding a lot of information, and so is losing power. However, imagine we are trying to decide which of two high jumpers is the better. They each jump over a bar at a fixed height, and then the height is increased. It is only when one fails to jump a given height and the other succeeds that a winner can be announced. It does not matter how many jumps both have cleared.

1 Snedecor GW, Cochran WG. In: *Statistical Methods*, 7th ed. Iowa: Iowa State University Press, 1980:47.
2 Cochran WG. Some methods for strengthening the common χ^2 tests. *Biometrics* 1956;**10**: 417–51.
3 Yates F. Contingency tables involving small numbers and the χ^2 test. *J Roy Stat Soc Suppl* 1934;**1**:217–35.
4 Capples ME, McKnight A. Randomised controlled trial of health promotions in general practice for patients at high cardiovascular risk. *BMJ* 1994;**309**:993–6.

Exercises

Exercise 8.1

In a trial of new drug against a standard drug for the treatment of depression the new drug caused some improvement in 56% of 73 patients and the standard drug some improvement in 41% of 70 patients. The results were assessed in five categories as follows:

New treatment: much improved 18, improved 23, unchanged 15, worse 9, much worse 8; Standard treatment: much improved 12, improved 17, unchanged 19, worse 13, much worse 9.

What is the value of X^2 which takes no account of the ordered value of data, what is the value of the X^2 test for trend, and the P value? How many degrees of freedom are there? What is the value of P in each case?

Exercise 8.2

An outbreak of pediculosis capitis is being investigated in a girls' school containing 291 pupils. Of 130 children who live in a nearby housing estate 18 were infested and of 161 who live elsewhere 37 were infested. What is the X^2 value of the difference, and what is its significance? Find the difference in infestation rates and a 95% confidence interval for the difference.

Exercise 8.3

The 55 affected girls were divided at random into two groups of 29 and 26. The first group received a standard local application and the second group a new local application. The efficacy of each was measured by clearance of the infestation after one application. By this measure the standard application failed in ten cases and the new application in five. What is the X^2 value of the difference (with Yates' correction), and what is its significance? What is the difference in clearance rates and an approximate 95% confidence interval?

Exercise 8.4

A general practitioner reviewed all patient notes in four practices for 1 year. Newly diagnosed cases of asthma were noted, and whether or not the case was referred to hospital. The following referrals were found (total cases in parentheses): practice A, 14 (103); practice B, 11 (92); practice C, 39 (166); practice D, 31 (221). What are the X^2 and P values for the distribution of the referrals in these practices? Do they suggest that any one practice has significantly more referrals than others?

9 Exact probability test

Sometimes in a comparison of the frequency of observations in a fourfold table the numbers are too small for the χ^2 test (Chapter 8). The exact probability test devised by Fisher, Irwin, and Yates[1] provides a way out of the difficulty. Tables based on it have been published—for example by Geigy[2]—showing levels at which the null hypothesis can be rejected. The method will be described here because, with the aid of a calculator, the exact probability is easily computed.

Consider the following circumstances. Some soldiers are being trained as parachutists. One rather windy afternoon 55 practice jumps take place at two localities, dropping zone A and dropping zone B. Of 15 men who jump at dropping zone A, five suffer sprained ankles, and of 40 who jump at dropping zone B, two suffer this injury. The casualty rate at dropping zone A seems unduly high, so the medical officer in charge decides to investigate the disparity. Is it a difference that might be expected by chance? If not it deserves deeper study. The figures are set out in Table 9.1. The null hypothesis is that there is no difference in the probability of injury generating the proportion of injured men at each dropping zone.

The method to be described tests the exact probability of observing the particular set of frequencies in the table if the marginal totals (that is, the totals in the last row and column) are kept at

Table 9.1   Numbers of men injured and uninjured in parachute training at two dropping zones

	Injured	Uninjured	Total
Dropping zone A	5	10	15
Dropping zone B	2	38	40
Total	7	48	55

their present values. But to the probability of getting this particular set of frequencies we have to add the probability of getting a set of frequencies showing greater disparity between the two dropping zones. This is because we are concerned to know the probability not only of the observed figures but also of the more extreme cases. This may seem obscure, but it ties in with the idea of calculating tail areas in the continuous case.

For convenience of computation the table is changed round to get the smallest number in the top left hand cell. We therefore begin by constructing Table 9.2 from Table 9.1 by transposing the upper and lower rows.

Table 9.2   Numbers in Table 9.1 rearranged for exact probability test

	Injured	Uninjured	Total
Dropping zone B	2	38	40
Dropping zone A	5	10	15
Total	7	48	55

The number of possible tables with these marginal totals is eight, that is, the smallest marginal total plus one. The eight sets are illustrated in Table 9.3. They are numbered in accordance with the top left hand cell. The figures in our example appear in set 2.

For the general case we can use the following notation:[1]

1st variable

		1	0	
2nd variable	1	a	b	r_1
	0	c	d	r_2
		s_1	s_2	N

Table 9.3   Sets of frequencies in Table 9.2 with same marginal totals

0	40	40		1	39	40
7	8	15		6	9	15
7	48	55		7	48	55
	Set 0				Set 1	
2	38	40		3	37	40
5	10	15		4	11	15
7	48	55		7	48	55
	Set 2				Set 3	
4	36	40		5	35	40
3	12	15		2	13	15
7	48	55		7	48	55
	Set 4				Set 5	
6	34	40		7	33	40
1	14	15		0	15	15
7	48	55		7	48	55
	Set 6				Set 7	

The exact probability for any table is now determined from the following formula:

$$\frac{r_1! \; r_2! \; s_1! \; s_2!}{N! \; a! \; b! \; c! \; d!}$$

The exclamation mark denotes "factorial" and means successive multiplication by cardinal numbers in descending series; for example 4! means $4 \times 3 \times 2 \times 1$. By convention $0! = 1$. Factorial functions are available on most calculators, but care is needed not to exceed the maximum number available on the calculator. Generally factorials can be cancelled out for easy computation on a calculator (see below).

With this formula we have to find the probability attached to the observations in Table 9.1, which is equivalent to Table 9.2, and is denoted by set 2 in Table 9.3. We also have to find the probabilities attached to the more extreme cases. If ad–bc is negative, then the extreme cases are obtained by progressively decreasing cells a and d and increasing b and c by the same amount. If $ad - bc$ is positive, then progressively *increase* cells a and d and decrease b and c by the same amount.[3] For Table 9.2 $ad - bc$ is negative and so the more extreme cases are sets 0 and 1.

The best way of doing this is to start with set 0. Call the probability attached to this set P_0. Then, applying the formula, we get:

$$P_0 = \frac{40! \ 15! \ 7! \ 48!}{55! \ 0! \ 40! \ 7! \ 8!}$$

This cancels down to

$$P_0 = \frac{15! \ 48!}{55! \ 8!}$$

For computation on a calculator the factorials can be cancelled out further by removing 8! from 15! and 48! from 55! to give

$$\frac{15 \times 14 \times 13 \times 12 \times 11 \times 10 \times 9}{55 \times 54 \times 53 \times 52 \times 51 \times 50 \times 49}$$

We now start from the left and divide and multiply alternately. However, on an eight digit calculator we would thereby obtain the result $0 \cdot 0000317$ which does not give enough significant figures. Consequently we first multiply the 15 by 1000. Alternate dividing and multiplying then gives $0 \cdot 0317107$. We continue to work with this figure, which is $P_0 \times 1000$, and we now enter it in the memory while also retaining it on the display.

Remembering that we are now working with units 1000 times larger than the real units, to calculate the probability for set 1 we take the value of P_0, multiply it by b and c from set 0, and divide it by a and d from set 1. That is

$$P_1 = P_0 \times \frac{(b_0 \times c_0)}{(a_1 \times d_1)} = 0 \cdot 0317107 \times \frac{(40 \times 7)}{(1 \times 9)}$$

$$= 0 \cdot 9865551.$$

The figure for P_1 is retained on the display.

Likewise, to calculate the probability for set 2:

$$P_2 = P_1 \times \frac{(b_1 \times c_1)}{(a_2 \times d_2)} = 0.9865551 \times \frac{(39 \times 6)}{(2 \times 10)}$$
$$= 11.542694.$$

This is as far as we need go, but for illustration we will calculate the probabilities for all possible tables for the given marginal totals.

Set	Probability
0	0·0000317
1	0·0009866
2	0·0115427
3	0·0664581
4	0·2049126
5	0·3404701
6	0·2837251
7	0·0918729
Total	0·9999998

A useful check is that all the probabilities should sum to one (within the limits of rounding).

The observed set has a probability of 0·0115427. The P value is the probability of getting the observed set, or *one more extreme*. A one tailed P value would be

$$0.0115427 + 0.0009866 + 0.0000317 = 0.01256$$

and this is the conventional approach. Armitage and Berry[1] favour the mid P value, which is

$$(0.5) \times 0.0115427 + 0.0009866 + 0.0000317 = 0.0068.$$

To get the two tailed value we double the one tailed result, thus $P = 0.025$ for the conventional or $P = 0.0136$ for the mid P approach. The conventional approach to calculating the P value for Fisher's exact test has been shown to be conservative (that is, it requires more evidence than is necessary to reject a false null hypothesis). The mid P is less conservative (that is more powerful) and also has some theoretical advantages. This is the one we advocate. For larger samples the P value obtained from a χ^2 test with Yates' correction will correspond to the conventional approach, and the P value from the uncorrected test will correspond to the mid P value.

In either case, the P value is less than the conventional 5% level; the medical officer can conclude that there is a problem in dropping zone A. The calculation of confidence intervals for the difference in proportions for small samples is complicated so we rely on the large sample formula given in Chapter 6. The way to present the results is: Injury rate in dropping zone A was 33%, in dropping zone B 5%; difference 28% (95% confidence interval 3·5 to 53·1% (from Chapter 6)), P = 0·0136 (Fisher's Exact test mid P).

Common questions

Why is Fisher's test called an exact test?

Because of the discrete nature of the data, and the limited amount of it, combinations of results which give the same marginal totals can be listed, and probabilities attached to them. Thus, given these marginal totals we can work out exactly what is the probability of getting an observed result, in the same way that we can work out exactly the probability of getting six heads out of ten tosses of a fair coin. One difficulty is that there may not be combinations which correspond "exactly" to 95%, so we cannot get an "exact" 95% confidence interval but (say) one with a 97% coverage or one with a 94% coverage.

1 Armitage P, Berry G. In: *Statistical Methods in Medical Research*. Oxford: Blackwell Scientific Publications, 1994:123–4.
2 Lentner C, ed. *Geigy Scientific Tables*, 8th ed. Basle: Geigy, 1982.
3 Strike PW. *Statistical Methods in Laboratory Medicine*. Oxford: Butterworth-Heinemann, 1991.

Exercises

Exercise 9.1

Of 30 men employed in a small workshop 18 worked in one department and 12 in another department. In one year five of the 18 reported sick with septic hands, and of the 12 men in the other department one did so. Is there a difference in the departments and how would you report this result?

10 Rank score tests

Population distributions are characterised, or defined, by parameters such as the mean and standard deviation. For skew distributions we would need to know other parameters such as the degree of skewness before the distribution could be identified uniquely, but the mean and standard deviation identify the Normal distribution uniquely. The t test described earlier depends for its validity on an assumption that the data originate from a Normally distributed population, and, when two groups are compared, the difference between the two samples arises simply because they differ only in their mean value. However, if we were concerned that the data did not originate from a Normally distributed population, then there are tests available which do not make use of this assumption. Because the data are no longer Normally distributed, the distribution cannot be characterised by a few parameters, and so the tests are often called "non-parametric". This is somewhat of a misnomer because, as we shall see, to be able to say anything useful about the population we must compare parameters. As was mentioned in Chapter 5, if the sample sizes in both groups are large lack of Normality is of less concern, and the large sample tests described in that chapter would apply.

Wilcoxon signed rank sum test

Wilcoxon and Mann and Whitney described rank sum tests,

which have been shown to be the same. Convention has now ascribed the Wilcoxon test to paired data and the Mann–Whitney U test to unpaired data.

Boogert et al.[1] (data also given in Shott[2]) used ultrasound to record fetal movements before and after chorionic villus sampling. The percentage of time the fetus spent moving is given in Table 10.1 for ten pregnant women.

Table 10.1 Wilcoxon test on fetal movement before and after chorionic villus sampling[1][2]

Patient no (1)	Before Sampling (2)	After Sampling (3)	Difference (before–after) (4)	Rank (5)	Signed rank (6)
1	25	18	7	9	9
2	24	27	−3	5·5	−5·5
3	28	25	3	5·5	5·5
4	15	20	−5	8	−8
5	20	17	3	5·5	5·5
6	23	24	−1	1·5	−1·5
7	21	24	−3	5·5	−5·5
8	20	22	−2	3	−3
9	20	19	1	1·5	1·5
10	27	19	8	10	10

If we are concerned that the differences in percentage of time spent moving are unlikely to be Normally distributed we could use the Wilcoxon signed rank test using the following assumptions:

1. The paired differences are independent.
2. The differences come from a symmetrical distribution.

We do not need to perform a test to ensure that the differences come from a symmetrical distribution: an "eyeball" test will suffice. A plot of the differences in column (4) of Table 10.1 is given in Figure 10.1 and shows that distribution of the differences is plausibly symmetrical. The differences are then ranked in column 5 (negative values are ignored and zero values omitted). When two or more differences are identical each is allotted the point half way between the ranks they would fill if distinct, irrespective of the plus or minus sign. For instance, the differences of − 1 (patient 6) and + 1 (patient 9) fill ranks 1 and 2. As $(1 + 2)/2 = 1·5$, they are allotted rank 1·5. In column (6) the ranks are repeated for column (5), but to each is attached the sign of the difference from column (4). A useful check is that the sum of the ranks must add to $n(n + 1)/2$. In this case $10(10 + 1)/2 = 55$.

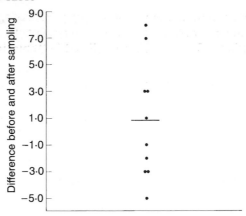

Figure 10.1   Plot of differences in fetal movement with mean value.[1]

The numbers representing the positive ranks and the negative ranks in column (6) are added up separately and only the smaller of the two totals is used. Irrespective of its sign, the total is referred to Table D (Appendix) against the number of pairs used in the investigation. Rank totals *larger* than those in the table are *non-*significant at the level of probability shown. In this case the smaller of the ranks is 23·5. This is larger than the number (8) given for ten pairs in Table D and so the result is not significant. A confidence interval for the interval is described by Campbell and Gardner[3] and Gardner and Altman,[4] and is easily obtained from the programs CIA[5] or MINITAB.[6] The median difference is zero. CIA gives the 95% confidence interval as −2·50 to 4·00. This is quite narrow and so from this small study we can conclude that we have little evidence that chorionic villus sampling alters the movement of the fetus.

Note, perhaps contrary to intuition, that the Wilcoxon test, although a rank test, may give a different value if the data are transformed, say by taking logarithms. Thus it may be worth plotting the distribution of the differences for a number of transformations to see if they make the distribution appear more symmetrical.

Unpaired samples

A senior registrar in the rheumatology clinic of a district hospital has designed a clinical trial of a new drug for rheumatoid arthritis.

Twenty patients were randomised into two groups of ten to receive either the standard therapy A or a new treatment, B. The plasma globulin fractions after treatment are listed in Table 10.2.

Table 10.2 Plasma globulin fraction after randomisation to treatments A or B

| Treatment A | 38 | 26 | 29 | 41 | 36 | 31 | 32 | 30 | 35 | 33 |
| Treatment B | 45 | 28 | 27 | 38 | 40 | 42 | 39 | 39 | 34 | 45 |

We wish to test whether the new treatment has changed the plasma globulin, and we are worried about the assumption of Normality.

The first step is to plot the data (Figure 10.2).

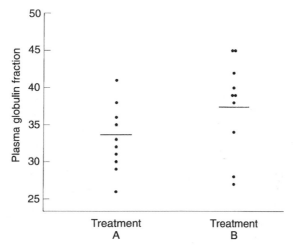

Figure 10.2 Plasma globulin fraction after treatments A or B with mean values.

The clinician was concerned about the lack of Normality of the underlying distribution of the data and so decided to use a non-parametric test. The appropriate test is the Mann–Whitney U test and is computed as follows.

The observations in the two samples are combined into a single series and ranked in order but in the ranking the figures from one sample must be distinguished from those of the other. The data appear as set out in Table 10.3. To save space they have been set out in two columns, but a single ranking is done. The figures for sample B are set in bold type. Again the sum of the ranks is $n(n+1)/2$.

Table 10.3   Combined results of Table 10.2

Globulin fraction	Rank	Globulin fraction	Rank
26	1	36	11
27	2	38	12·5
28	3	38	12·5
29	4	39	14·5
30	5	39	14·5
31	6	40	16
32	7	41	17
33	8	42	18
34	9	45	19·5
35	10	45	19·5

Totals of ranks: sample A, 81·5; sample B, 128·5

The ranks for the two samples are now added separately, and the smaller total is used. It is referred to Table E (Appendix), with n_1 equal to the number of observations in one sample and n_2 equal to the number of observations in the other sample. In this case they both equal 10. At $n_1 = 10$ and $n_2 = 10$ the upper part of the table shows the figure 78. The smaller total of the ranks is 81·5. Since this is slightly larger than 78 it does not reach the 5% level of probability. The result is therefore not significant at that level. In the lower part of Table E, which gives the figures for the 1% level of probability, the figure for $n_1 = 10$ and $n_2 = 10$ is 71. As expected, the result is further from that than the 5% figure of 78.

To calculate a meaningful confidence interval we assume that if the two samples come from different populations the distribution of these populations differs only in that one appears shifted to the left or right of the other. This means, for example, that we do not expect one sample to be strongly right skewed and one to be strongly left skewed. If the assumption is reasonable then a confidence interval for the median difference can be calculated.[34] Note that the computer program does not calculate the difference in medians, but rather the median of all possible differences between the two samples. This is usually close to the median difference and has theoretical advantages. From CIA we find that the difference in medians is $-5·5$ and the approximate 95% confidence interval is -10 to $1·0$. As might be expected from the significance test this

96

interval includes zero. Although this result is not significant it would be unwise to conclude that there was no evidence that treatments A and B differed because the confidence interval is quite wide. This suggests that a larger study should be planned.

If the two samples are of unequal size a further calculation is needed after the ranking has been carried out as in Table 10.3.

Let n_1 = number of patients or objects in the smaller sample and T_1 the total of the ranks for that sample. Let n_2 = number of patients or objects in the larger sample. Then calculate T_2 from the following formula:

$$T_2 = n_1(n_1 + n_2 + 1) - T_1.$$

Finally enter Table E with the smaller of T_1 or T_2. As before, only totals smaller than the critical points in Table E are significant. See Exercise 10.2 for an example of this method.

If there are only a few ties, that is if two or more values in the data are equal (say less than 10% of the data) then for sample sizes outside the range of Table E we can calculate

$$z = \frac{|T_1 - n_1(n_1 + n_2 + 1)/2|}{\sqrt{[n_1 n_2 (n_1 + n_2 + 1)/12]}}.$$

On the null hypothesis that the two samples come from the same population, z is approximately Normally distributed, mean zero and standard deviation one, and can be referred to Table A (Appendix) to calculate the P value.

From the data of Table 10.2 we obtain

$$z = \frac{|81 \cdot 5 - 10 \times 21/2|}{\sqrt{(10 \times 10 \times 21/12)}} = 1 \cdot 78$$

and from Table A we find that P is about 0·075, which corroborates the earlier result.

The advantages of these tests based on ranking are that they can be safely used on data that are not at all Normally distributed, that they are quick to carry out, and that no calculator is needed. Non-Normally distributed data can sometimes be transformed by the use of logarithms or some other method to make them Normally distributed, and a *t* test performed. Consequently the best procedure

97

to adopt may require careful thought. The extent and nature of the difference between two samples is often brought out more clearly by standard deviations and t tests than by non-parametric tests.

Common questions

Non-parametric tests are valid for both non-Normally distributed data and Normally distributed data, so why not use them all the time?

It would seem prudent to use non-parametric tests in all cases, which would save one the bother of testing for Normality. Parametric tests are preferred, however, for the following reasons:

1. As I have tried to emphasise in this book, we are rarely interested in a significance test alone; we would like to say something about the population from which the samples came, and this is best done with estimates of parameters and confidence intervals.
2. It is difficult to do flexible modelling with non-parametric tests, for example allowing for confounding factors using multiple regression (see Chapter 11).

Do non-parametric tests compare medians?

It is a commonly held belief that a Mann–Whitney U test is in fact a test for differences in medians. However, two groups could have the same median and yet have a significant Mann–Whitney U test. Consider the following data for two groups, each with 100 observations. Group 1: 98 (0), 1, 2; Group 2: 51 (0), 1, 48 (2). The median in both cases is 0, but from the Mann–Whitney test $P<0.0001$.

Only if we are prepared to make the additional assumption that the difference in the two groups is simply a shift in location (that is, the distribution of the data in one group is simply shifted by a fixed amount from the other) can we say that the test is a test of the difference in medians. However, if the groups have the same distribution, then a shift in location will move medians and means by the same amount and so the difference in medians is the same as the difference in means. Thus the Mann–Whitney U test is also a test for the difference in means.

How is the Mann–Whitney U test related to the t test?

If one were to input the ranks of the data rather than the data themselves into a two sample t test program, the P value obtained would be very close to that produced by a Mann–Whitney U test.

1 Boogert A, Manhigh A, Visser GHA. The immediate effects of chronic villus sampling on fetal movements. *Am J Obstet Gynecol* 1987;**157**:137–9.
2 Shott S. *Statistics for Health Professionals.* Philadelphia: WB Saunders, 1990.
3 Campbell MJ, Gardner MJ. Calculating confidence intervals for some non-parametric analyses. *BMJ* 1988;**296**:1369–71.
4 Gardner MJ, Altman DG. *Statistics with Confidence. Confidence Intervals and Statistical Guidelines.* London: BMJ Publishing Group, 1989.
5 Gardner MJ, Gardner SB, Winter PD. *CIA (Confidence Interval Analysis).* London: BMJ Publishing Group, 1989.
6 Ryan BF, Joiner BL, Ryan TA. *Minitab Handbook*, 2nd ed. Boston: Duxbury Press, 1985.

Exercises

Exercise 10.1

A new treatment in the form of tablets for the prophylaxis of migraine has been introduced, to be taken before an impending attack. Twelve patients agree to try this remedy in addition to the usual general measures they take, subject to advice from their doctor on the taking of analgesics also.

A crossover trial with identical placebo tablets is carried out over a period of 8 months. The numbers of attacks experienced by each patient on, first, the new treatment and, secondly, the placebo were as follows: patient (1) 4 and 2; patient (2) 12 and 6; patient (3) 6 and 6; patient (4) 3 and 5; patient (5) 15 and 9; patient (6) 10 and 11; patient (7) 2 and 4; patient (8) 5 and 6; patient (9) 11 and 3; patient (10) 4 and 7; patient (11) 6 and 0; patient (12) 2 and 5. In a Wilcoxon rank sum test what is the smaller total of ranks? Is it significant at the 5% level?

Exercise 10.2

Another doctor carried out a similar pilot study with this preparation on 12 patients, giving the same placebo to ten other patients. The numbers of migraine attacks experienced by the patients over a period of 6 months were as follows.

Group receiving new preparation: patient (1) 8; (2) 6; (3) 0; (4) 3; (5) 14; (6) 5; (7) 11; (8) 2

Group receiving placebo: patient (9) 7; (10) 10; (11) 4; (12) 11; (13) 2; (14) 8; (15) 8; (16) 6; (17) 1; (18) 5.

In a Mann–Whitney two sample test what is the smaller total of ranks? Which sample of patients provides it? Is the difference significant at the 5% level?

11 Correlation and regression

The word *correlation* is used in everyday life to denote some form of association. We might say that we have noticed a correlation between foggy days and attacks of wheeziness. However, in statistical terms we use correlation to denote association between two quantitative variables. We also assume that the association is *linear*, that one variable increases or decreases a fixed amount for a unit increase or decrease in the other. The other technique that is often used in these circumstances is *regression*, which involves estimating the best straight line to summarise the association.

Correlation coefficient

The degree of association is measured by a correlation coefficient, denoted by r. It is sometimes called Pearson's correlation coefficient after its originator and is a measure of linear association. If a curved line is needed to express the relationship, other and more complicated measures of the correlation must be used.

The correlation coefficient is measured on a scale that varies from $+1$ through 0 to -1. Complete correlation between two variables is expressed by either $+1$ or -1. When one variable increases as the other increases the correlation is positive; when one decreases as the other increases it is negative. Complete absence

100

of correlation is represented by 0. Figure 11.1 gives some graphical representations of correlation.

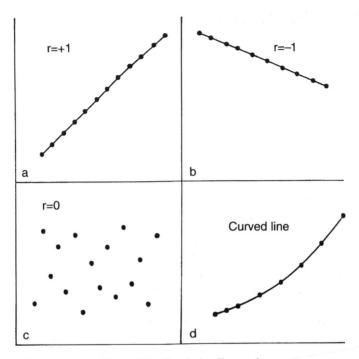

Figure 11.1   Correlation illustrated.

Looking at data: scatter diagrams

When an investigator has collected two series of observations and wishes to see whether there is a relationship between them, he or she should first construct a scatter diagram. The vertical scale represents one set of measurements and the horizontal scale the other. If one set of observations consists of experimental results and the other consists of a time scale or observed classification of some kind, it is usual to put the experimental results on the vertical axis. These represent what is called the "dependent variable". The "independent variable", such as time or height or some other observed classification, is measured along the horizontal axis, or baseline.

101

The words "independent" and "dependent" could puzzle the beginner because it is sometimes not clear what is dependent on what. This confusion is a triumph of common sense over misleading terminology, because often each variable is dependent on some third variable, which may or may not be mentioned. It is reasonable, for instance, to think of the height of children as dependent on age rather than the converse but consider a positive correlation between mean tar yield and nicotine yield of certain brands of cigarette.[1] The nicotine liberated is unlikely to have its origin in the tar: both vary in parallel with some other factor or factors in the composition of the cigarettes. The yield of the one does not seem to be "dependent" on the other in the sense that, on average, the height of a child depends on his age. In such cases it often does not matter which scale is put on which axis of the scatter diagram. However, if the intention is to make inferences about one variable from the other, the observations *from which* the inferences are to be made are usually put on the baseline. As a further example, a plot of monthly deaths from heart disease against monthly sales of ice cream would show a negative association. However, it is hardly likely that eating ice cream protects from heart disease! It is simply that the mortality rate from heart disease is inversely related—and ice cream consumption positively related—to a third factor, namely environmental temperature.

Calculation of the correlation coefficient

A paediatric registrar has measured the pulmonary anatomical dead space (in ml) and height (in cm) of 15 children. The data are given in Table 11.1 and the scatter diagram shown in Figure 11.2. Each dot represents one child, and it is placed at the point corresponding to the measurement of the height (horizontal axis) and the dead space (vertical axis). The registrar now inspects the pattern to see whether it seems likely that the area covered by the dots centres on a straight line or whether a curved line is needed. In this case the paediatrician decides that a straight line can adequately describe the general trend of the dots. His next step will therefore be to calculate the correlation coefficient.

When making the scatter diagram (Figure 11.2) to show the heights and pulmonary anatomical dead spaces in the 15 children, the paediatrician set out figures as in columns (1), (2), and (3) of

Table 11.1   *Correlation between height and pulmonary anatomical dead space in 15 children*

Child number (1)	Height (cm) (2)	Dead space (ml), y (3)
1	110	44
2	116	31
3	124	43
4	129	45
5	131	56
6	138	79
7	142	57
8	150	56
9	153	58
10	155	92
11	156	78
12	159	64
13	164	88
14	168	112
15	174	101
Total	2169	1004
Mean	144·6	66·933

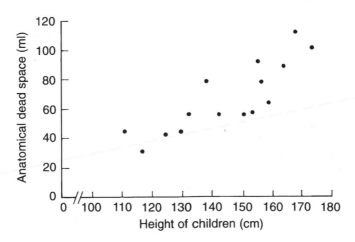

Figure 11.2   *Scatter diagram of relation in 15 children between height and pulmonary anatomical dead space.*

Table 11.1. It is helpful to arrange the observations in serial order of the independent variable when one of the two variables is clearly identifiable as independent. The corresponding figures for the dependent variable can then be examined in relation to the

103

increasing series for the independent variable. In this way we get the same picture, but in numerical form, as appears in the scatter diagram.

The calculation of the correlation coefficient is as follows, with x representing the values of the independent variable (in this case height) and y representing the values of the dependent variable (in this case anatomical dead space). The formula to be used is:

$$r = \frac{\Sigma(x-\bar{x})(y-\bar{y})}{\sqrt{[\Sigma(x-\bar{x})^2(y-\bar{y})^2]}}$$

which can be shown to be equal to:

$$r = \frac{\Sigma xy - \bar{n}\bar{x}\bar{y}}{(n-1)SD(x)SD(y)}.$$

Calculator procedure

Find the mean and standard deviation of x, as described in Chapter 2: $\bar{x}$, SD(x).

$$\bar{x} = 144{\cdot}6, \; SD(x) = 19{\cdot}3679$$

Find the mean and standard deviation of y: $\bar{y}$, SD(y).

$$\bar{y} = 66{\cdot}93, \; SD(y) = 23{\cdot}6476$$

Subtract 1 from n and multiply by SD(x) and SD(y), (n − 1)SD(x)SD(y)

$$14 \times 19{\cdot}3679 \times 23{\cdot}6976 \; (6412{\cdot}0609)$$

This gives us the denominator of the formula. (Remember to exit from "Stat" mode.)

For the numerator multiply each value of x by the corresponding value of y, add these values together and store them.

$$110 \times 44 = \mathbf{Min}$$

$$116 \times 31 = \mathbf{M+}$$

etc.

This stores Σxy (150605) in memory. Subtract $n\bar{x}\bar{y}$.

$$\mathbf{MR} - 15 \times 144\cdot6 \times 66\cdot93 \ (5426\cdot6)$$

Finally divide the numerator by the denominator.

$$r = 5426\cdot6/6412\cdot0609 = 0\cdot846.$$

The correlation coefficient of $0\cdot846$ indicates a strong positive correlation between size of pulmonary anatomical dead space and height of child. But in interpreting correlation it is important to remember that *correlation is not causation*. There may or may not be a causative connection between the two correlated variables. Moreover, if there *is* a connection it may be indirect.

A part of the variation in one of the variables (as measured by its variance) can be thought of as being due to its relationship with the other variable and another part as due to undetermined (often "random") causes. The part due to the dependence of one variable on the other is measured by r^2. For these data $r^2 = 0\cdot716$, so we can say that 72% of the variation between children in size of the anatomical dead space is accounted for by the height of the child. If we wish to label the strength of the association, for absolute values of r, $0-0\cdot19$ is regarded as very weak, $0\cdot2-0\cdot39$ as weak, $0\cdot40-0\cdot59$ as moderate, $0\cdot6-0\cdot79$ as strong and $0\cdot8-1$ as very strong correlation, but these are rather arbitrary limits, and the context of the results should be considered.

Significance test

To test whether the association is merely apparent, and might have arisen by chance use the *t* test in the following calculation:

$$t = r \sqrt{\frac{n-2}{1-r^2}}. \qquad (11.1)$$

The *t* table (Appendix, Table B) is entered at $n-2$ degrees of freedom.

For example, the correlation coefficient for these data was $0\cdot846$.

The number of pairs of observations was 15. Applying equation 11.1, we have:

$$t = 0 \cdot 846 \sqrt{\frac{15 - 2}{1 - 0 \cdot 846^2}} = 5 \cdot 72.$$

Entering Table B at $15 - 2 = 13$ degrees of freedom we find that at $t = 5 \cdot 72$, $P < 0 \cdot 001$, so the correlation coefficient may be regarded as highly significant. Thus (as could be seen immediately from the scatter plot) we have a very strong correlation between dead space and height which is most unlikely to have arisen by chance.

The assumptions governing this test are:

1. That both variables are plausibly Normally distributed.
2. That there is a linear relationship between them.
3. The null hypothesis is that there is no association between them.

The test should not be used for comparing two methods of measuring the same quantity, such as two methods of measuring peak expiratory flow rate. Its use in this way appears to be a common mistake, with a significant result being interpreted as meaning that one method is equivalent to the other. The reasons have been extensively discussed[2] but it is worth recalling that a significant result tells us little about the strength of a relationship. From the formula it should be clear that with even with a very weak relationship (say $r = 0 \cdot 1$) we would get a significant result with a large enough sample (say n over 1000).

Spearman rank correlation

A plot of the data may reveal outlying points well away from the main body of the data, which could unduly influence the calculation of the correlation coefficient. Alternatively the variables may be quantitative discrete such as a mole count, or ordered categorical such as a pain score. A non-parametric procedure, due to Spearman, is to replace the observations by their ranks in the calculation of the correlation coefficient.

This results in a simple formula for Spearman's rank correlation, r_s.

$$r_s = 1 - \frac{6 \Sigma d^2}{n(n^2 - 1)}$$

where d is the difference in the ranks of the two variables for a given individual. Thus we can derive Table 11.2 from the data in Table 11.1.

Table 11.2 Derivation of Spearman rank correlation from data of Table 11.1

Child number	Rank height	Rank dead space	d	d^2
1	1	3	2	4
2	2	1	−1	1
3	3	2	−1	1
4	4	4	0	0
5	5	5·5	0·5	0·25
6	6	11	5	25
7	7	7	0	0
8	8	5·5	−2·5	6·25
9	9	8	−1	1
10	10	13	3	9
11	11	10	−1	1
12	12	9	−3	9
13	13	12	−1	1
14	14	15	1	1
15	15	14	−1	1
Total				60·5

From this we get that

$$r_s = 1 - \frac{6 \times 60 \cdot 5}{15 \times (225 - 1)} = 0 \cdot 8920.$$

In this case the value is very close to that of the Pearson correlation coefficient. For n>10, the Spearman rank correlation coefficient can be tested for significance using the t test given earlier.

The regression equation

Correlation describes the strength of an association between two variables, and is completely symmetrical, the correlation between A and B is the same as the correlation between B and A. However, if the two variables are related it means that when one changes by a certain amount the other changes on an average by a certain amount. For instance, in the children described earlier greater height is associated, on average, with greater anatomical dead space. If y represents the dependent variable and x the independent variable, this relationship is described as the regression of y on x.

The relationship can be represented by a simple equation called the regression equation. In this context "regression" (the term is a historical anomaly) simply means that the average value of y is a "function" of x, that is, it changes with x.

The regression equation representing how much y changes with any given change of x can be used to construct a *regression line* on a scatter diagram, and in the simplest case this is assumed to be a straight line. The direction in which the line slopes depends on whether the correlation is positive or negative. When the two sets of observations increase or decrease together (positive) the line slopes upwards from left to right; when one set decreases as the other increases the line slopes downwards from left to right. As the line must be straight, it will probably pass through few, if any, of the dots. Given that the association is well described by a straight line we have to define two features of the line if we are to place it correctly on the diagram. The first of these is its distance above the baseline; the second is its slope. They are expressed in the following *regression equation*:

$$y = \alpha + \beta x.$$

With this equation we can find a series of values of y_{fit}, the variable, that correspond to each of a series of values of x, the independent variable. The parameters α and β have to be estimated from the data. The parameter α signifies the distance above the baseline at which the regression line cuts the vertical (y) axis; that is, when $y = 0$. The parameter β (the *regression coefficient*) signifies the amount by which change in x must be multiplied to give the corresponding average change in y, or the amount y changes for a unit increase in x. In this way it represents the degree to which the line slopes upwards or downwards.

The regression equation is often more useful than the correlation coefficient. It enables us to predict y from x and gives us a better summary of the relationship between the two variables. If, for a particular value of x, x_i, the regression equation predicts a value of y_{fit}, the prediction error is $y_i - y_{fit}$. It can easily be shown that *any* straight line passing through the mean values $\bar{x}$ and $\bar{y}$ will give a total prediction error $\Sigma(y_i - y_{fit})$ of zero because the positive and negative terms exactly cancel. To remove the negative signs we square the differences and the regression equation chosen to minimise the sum of squares of the prediction errors, $S^2 = \Sigma(y - y_{fit})^2$.

108

We denote the sample estimates of α and β by a and b. It can be shown that the one straight line that minimises S^2, the *least squares estimate*, is given by

$$b = \frac{\Sigma(x - \bar{x})(y - \bar{y})}{\Sigma(x - \bar{x})^2}$$

and

$$a = \bar{y} - b\bar{x}.$$

It can be shown that

$$b = \frac{\Sigma xy - n\bar{x}\bar{y}}{(n-1)SD(x)^2} \qquad (11.2)$$

which is of use because we have calculated all the components of equation (11.2) in the calculation of the correlation coefficient.

The calculation of the correlation coefficient on the data in Table 11.1 gave the following:

$\Sigma xy = 150605$, $SD(x) = 19 \cdot 3679$, $\bar{y} = 66 \cdot 93$, $\bar{x} = 144 \cdot 6$.

Applying these figures to the formulae for the regression coefficients, we have:

$$b = \frac{150605 - 15 \times 66 \cdot 93 \times 144 \cdot 6}{14 \times 19 \cdot 3679^2} = \frac{5426 \cdot 6}{5251 \cdot 6}$$

$$= 1 \cdot 033 \text{ ml/cm}$$

$$a = 66 \cdot 93 - (1 \cdot 033 \times 144 \cdot 6) = -82 \cdot 4.$$

Therefore, in this case, the equation for the regression of y on x becomes

$$y = -82 \cdot 4 + 1 \cdot 033x.$$

This means that, on average, for every increase in height of 1 cm the increase in anatomical dead space is $1 \cdot 033$ ml *over the range of measurements made.*

The line representing the equation is shown superimposed on the scatter diagram of the data in Figure 11.3. The way to draw

109

the line is to take three values of x, one on the left side of the scatter diagram, one in the middle and one on the right, and substitute these in the equation, as follows:

If x = 110, y = (1·033 × 110) − 82·4 = 31·2

If x = 140, y = (1·033 × 140) − 82·4 = 62·2

If x = 170, y = (1·033 × 170) − 82·4 = 93·2.

Although two points are enough to define the line, three are better as a check. Having put them on a scatter diagram, we simply draw the line through them.

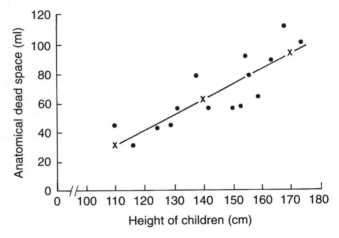

Figure 11.3 Regression line drawn on scatter diagram relating height and pulmonary anatomical dead space in 15 children (Figure 11.2).

The standard error of the slope SE(b) is given by:

$$SE(b) = \frac{S_{res}}{\sqrt{\Sigma(x - \bar{x})^2}} \qquad (11.3)$$

where S_{res} is the residual standard deviation, given by:

$$S_{res} = \sqrt{\frac{\Sigma(y - y_{fit})^2}{n - 2}}$$

This can be shown to be algebraically equal to $\sqrt{(SD(y)^2(1-r^2)(n-1)/(n-2))}$.

We already have to hand all of the terms in this expression. Thus S_{res} is the square root of $23 \cdot 6476^2(1-0 \cdot 846^2)14/13 = \sqrt{171 \cdot 2029} = 13 \cdot 08445$. The denominator of (11.3) is $72 \cdot 4680$.

Thus $SE(b) = 13 \cdot 08445/72 \cdot 4680 = 0 \cdot 18055$.

We can test whether the slope is significantly different from zero by:

$$t = b/SE(b) = 1 \cdot 033/0 \cdot 18055 = 5 \cdot 72.$$

Again, this has $n - 2 = 15 - 2 = 13$ degrees of freedom.

The assumptions governing this test are:

1. That the prediction errors are approximately Normally distributed. Note this does *not* mean that the x or y variables have to be Normally distributed.
2. That the relationship between the two variables is linear.
3. That the scatter of points about the line is approximately constant—we would not wish the variability of the dependent variable to be growing as the independent variable increases. If this is the case try taking logarithms of both the x and y variables.

Note that the test of significance for the slope gives exactly the same value of P as the test of significance for the correlation coefficient. Although the two tests are derived differently, they are algebraically equivalent, which makes intuitive sense.

We can obtain a 95% confidence interval for b from

$$b - t_{0 \cdot 05} \times SE(b) \text{ to } b + t_{0 \cdot 05} \times SE(b)$$

where the *t* statistic from Table B has 13 degrees of freedom, and is equal to $2 \cdot 160$.

Thus the 95% confidence interval is

$$1 \cdot 033 - 2 \cdot 160 \times 0 \cdot 18055 \text{ to } 1 \cdot 033 + 2 \cdot 160 \times 0 \cdot 18055$$
$$= 0 \cdot 643 \text{ to } 1 \cdot 422.$$

Regression lines give us useful information about the data they are collected from. They show how one variable changes on average with another, and they can be used to find out what one variable is likely to be when we know the other—provided that we ask this question within the limits of the scatter diagram. To project the line at either end—to extrapolate—is always risky because the

111

relationship between x and y may change or some kind of cut off point may exist. For instance, a regression line might be drawn relating the chronological age of some children to their bone age, and it might be a straight line between, say, the ages of 5 and 10 years, but to project it up to the age of 30 would clearly lead to error. Computer packages will often produce the intercept from a regression equation, with no warning that it may be totally meaningless. Consider a regression of blood pressure against age in middle aged men. The regression coefficient is often positive, indicating that blood pressure increases with age. The intercept is often close to zero, but it would be wrong to conclude that this is a reliable estimate of the blood pressure in newly born male infants!

More advanced methods

More than one independent variable is possible—in such a case the method is known as *multiple regression*.[34] This is the most versatile of statistical methods and can be used in many situations. Examples include: to allow for more than one predictor, age as well as height in the above example; to allow for covariates—in a clinical trial the dependent variable may be outcome after treatment, the first independent variable can be binary, 0 for placebo and 1 for active treatment and the second independent variable may be a baseline variable, measured before treatment, but likely to affect outcome.

Common questions

If two variables are correlated are they causally related?

It is a common error to confuse correlation and causation. All that correlation shows is that the two variables are associated. There may be a third variable, a *confounding* variable that is related to both of them. For example, monthly deaths by drowning and monthly sales of ice-cream are positively correlated, but no-one would say the relationship was causal!

How do I test the assumptions underlying linear regression?

Firstly always look at the scatter plot and ask, is it linear? Having obtained the regression equation, calculate the residuals $e_i = y_i - y_{fit}$. A histogram of e_i will reveal departures from Normality and a plot of e_i versus y_{fit} will reveal whether the residuals increase in size as y_{fit} increases.

1 Russell MAH, Cole PY, Idle MS, Adams L. Carbon monoxide yields of cigarettes and their relation to nicotine yield and type of filter. *BMJ* 1975;3:71–3.
2 Bland JM, Altman DG. Statistical methods for assessing agreement between two methods of clinical measurement. *Lancet* 1986;i:307–10.
3 Brown RA, Swanson-Beck J. *Medical Statistics on Personal Computers*, 2nd edn. London: BMJ Publishing Group, 1993.
4 Armitage P, Berry G. In: *Statistical Methods in Medical Research*, 3rd edn. Oxford: Blackwell Scientific Publications, 1994:312–41.

Exercises

Exercise 11.1

A study was carried out into the attendance rate at a hospital of people in 16 different geographical areas, over a fixed period of time. The distance of the centre from the hospital of each area was measured in miles. The results were as follows:

(1) 21%, 6·8; (2) 12%, 10·3; (3) 30%, 1·7; (4) 8%, 14·2; (5) 10%, 8·8; (6) 26%, 5·8; (7) 42%, 2·1; (8) 31%, 3·3; (9) 21%, 4·3; (10) 15%, 9·0; (11) 19%, 3·2; (12) 6%, 12·7; (13) 18%, 8·2; (14) 12%, 7·0; (15) 23%, 5·1; (16) 34%, 4·1.

What is the correlation coefficient between the attendance rate and mean distance of the geographical area?

Exercise 11.2

Find the Spearman rank correlation for the data given in Exercise 11.1.

Exercise 11.3

If the values of x from the data in Exercise 11.1 represent mean distance of the area from the hospital and values of y represent attendance rates, what is the equation for the regression of y on x? What does it mean?

Exercise 11.4

Find the standard error and 95% confidence interval for the slope.

12 Survival analysis

Survival analysis is concerned with studying the time between entry to a study and a subsequent event. Originally the analysis was concerned with time from treatment until death, hence the name, but survival analysis is applicable to many areas as well as mortality. Recent examples include time to discontinuation of a contraceptive, maximum dose of bronchoconstrictor required to reduce a patient's lung function to 80% of baseline, time taken to exercise to maximum tolerance, time that a transdermal patch can be left in place, time for a leg fracture to heal.

When the outcome of a study is the time between one event and another, a number of problems can occur.

1. The times are most unlikely to be Normally distributed.
2. We cannot afford to wait until events have happened to all the subjects, for example until all are dead. Some patients might have left the study early—they are *lost to follow up*. Thus the only information we have about some patients is that they were still alive at the last follow up. These are termed *censored observations*.

Kaplan–Meier survival curve

We look at the data using a Kaplan–Meier survival curve.[1]

Suppose that the survival times, including censored observations, after entry into the study (ordered by increasing duration) of a group

114

of n subjects are t_1, t_2, ... t_n. The proportion of subjects, $S(t)$, surviving beyond any follow up time (t_p) is estimated by

$$S(t) = \frac{(r_1 - d_1)}{r_1} \times \frac{(r_2 - d_2)}{r_2} \cdots \times \cdots \frac{r_p - d_p}{r_p}$$

where t_p is the largest survival time less than or equal to t and r_i is the number of subjects alive just before time t_i (the ith ordered survival time), d_i denotes the number who died at time t_i where i can be any value between 1 and p. For censored observations $d_i = 0$.

Method

Order the survival time by increasing duration starting with the shortest one. At each event (i) work out the number alive immediately before the event (r_i). Before the first event all the patients are alive and so $S(t) = 1$. If we denote the start of the study as t_0, where $t_0 = 0$, then we have $S(t_0) = 1$. We can now calculate the survival times t_i, for each value of i from 1 to n by means of the following recurrence formula.

Given the number of events (deaths), d_i, at time t_i and the number alive, r_i, just before t_i calculate

$$S(t_i) = \frac{r_i - d_i}{r_i} \times S(t_{i-1}).$$

We do this only for the events and not for censored observations. The survival curve is unchanged at the time of a censored observation, but at the next event after the censored observation the number of people "at risk" is reduced by the number censored between the two events.

Example of calculation of survival curve

McIllmurray and Turkie[2] describe a clinical trial of 69 patients for the treatment of Dukes' C colorectal cancer. The data for the two treatments, γ linoleic acid or control are given in Table 12.1.[23]

Table 12.1 *Survival in 49 patients with Dukes' C colorectal cancer, randomly assigned to either γ linoleic acid or control treatment*

Treatment	Survival time (months)
γ linoleic acid (n = 25)	1+, 5+, 6, 6, 9+, 10, 10, 10+, 12, 12, 12, 12, 12+, 13+, 15+, 16+, 20+, 24, 24+, 27+, 32, 34+, 36+, 36+, 44+
Control (n = 24)	3+, 6, 6, 6, 6, 8, 8, 12, 12, 12+, 15+, 16+, 18+, 18+, 20, 22+, 24, 28+, 28+, 28+, 30, 30+, 33+, 42

The calculation of the Kaplan–Meier survival curve for the 25 patients randomly assigned to receive γ linoleic acid is described in Table 12.2. The + sign indicates censored data. Until 6 months after treatment, there are no deaths, so $S(t) = 1$. The effect of the censoring is to remove from the alive group those that are censored. At time 6 months two subjects have been censored and so the number alive just before 6 months is 23. There are two deaths at 6 months.

Thus,

$$S(6) = \frac{1 \times (23-2)}{23} = 0.9130.$$

We now reduce the number alive ("at risk") by two. The censored event at 9 months reduces the "at risk" set to 20. At 10 months there are two deaths, so the proportion surviving is $18/20 = 0.90$ and the cumulative proportion surviving is $0.913 \times 0.90 = 0.8217$. The cumulative survival is conveniently stored in the memory of a calculator. As one can see the effect of the censored observations is to reduce the number at risk without affecting the survival curve $S(t)$.

Finally we plot the survival curve, as shown in Figure 12.1. The censored observations are shown as ticks on the line.

Log rank test

To compare two survival curves produced from two groups A and B we use the rather curiously named log rank test,[1] so called because it can be shown to be related to a test that uses the logarithms of the ranks of the data.

116

Table 12.2   Calculation of survival case for 25 patients randomly assigned to receive γ linoleic acid

Case (i)	Survival time (months) (t_i)	Number alive (r_i)	Deaths (d_i)	Proportion surviving $(r_i - d_i)/n_i$	Cumulative proportion surviving $S(t)$
	0	0	0	—	1
1	1 +	25	0	1	1
2	5 +	24	0	1	1
3	6	23	2	0·9130	0·9130
4	6				
5	9 +	21	0	1	0·9130
6	10	20	2	0·90	0·8217
7	10				
8	10 +				
9	12	17	4	0·7647	0·6284
10	12				
11	12				
12	12				
13	12 +				
14	13 +	12	0	1	0·6284
15	15 +	11	0	1	0·6284
16	16 +	10	0	1	0·6284
17	20 +	9	0	1	0·6284
18	24	8	1	0·875	0·5498
19	24 +				
20	27 +	6	0	1	0·5498
21	32	5	1	0·80	0·4399
22	34 +				
23	36 +				
24	36 +				
25	44 +				

The assumptions used in this test are:

1. That the survival times are ordinal or continuous.
2. That the risk of an event in one group relative to the other does not change with time. Thus if linoleic acid reduces the risk of death in patients with colorectal cancer, then this risk reduction does not change with time (the so called *proportional hazards assumption*).

We first order the data for the two groups combined, as shown in Table 12.3. As for the Kaplan–Meier survival curve, we now consider each event in turn, starting at time $t = 0$.

At each event (death) at time t_i we consider the total number alive (r_i) and the total number still alive in group A (r_{Ai}) up to that

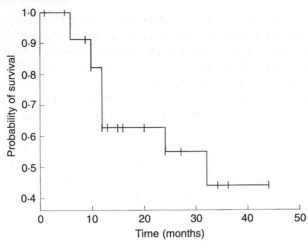

Figure 12.1   Survival curve of 25 patients with Dukes' C colorectal cancer treated with γ linoleic acid.

point. If we had a total of d_i events at time t_i, then, under the null hypothesis, we consider what proportion of these would have been expected in group A. Clearly the more people at risk in one group the more deaths (under the null hypothesis) we would expect.

Thus we obtain

$$E_{Ai} = r_{Ai}/r_i \times d_i.$$

The effect of the censored observations is to reduce the numbers at risk, but they do not contribute to the expected numbers.

Finally, we add the total number of expected events in group A, $E_A = \Sigma E_{Ai}$. If the total number of events in group B is E_B, we can deduce E_B from $E_B = n - E_A$. We do not calculate the expected number beyond the last event, in this case at time 42 months. Also, we would stop calculating the expected values if any survival times greater than the point we were at were found in one group only.

Finally, to test the null hypothesis of equal risk in the two groups we compute

$$X^2 = (O_A - E_A)^2/E_A + (O_B - E_B)^2/E_B$$

where O_A and O_B are the total number of events in groups A and B. We compare X^2 to a χ^2 distribution with one degree of freedom (one, because we have two groups and one constraint, namely that the total expected events must equal the total observed).

The calculation for the colorectal data is given in Table 12.3. The first non-censored event occurs at 6 months, at which there are six of them. By that time 46 patients are at risk, of whom 23 are in group A. Thus we would expect $6 \times 23/46 = 3$ to be in group A. At 8 months we have $46 - 6 = 40$ patients at risk of whom $23 - 2 = 21$ are in group A. There are two events, of which we would expect $2 \times 21/40 = 1.05$ to occur in group A.

The total expected number of events in A is $E_A = 11.3745$. The total number of events is 22, $O_A = 10$, $O_B = 12$. Thus $E_B = 10.6255$. Thus

$$X^2 = \frac{(10 - 11.37)^2}{11.37} + \frac{(12 - 10.63)^2}{10.63} = 0.34.$$

We compare this with the χ^2 table given in the appendix (Table C), to find that $P > 0.10$.

The relative risk can be estimated by $r = (O_A/E_A)/(O_B/E_B)$. The standard error of the log risk is given by[4]

$$SE(\log(r)) = \sqrt{(1/E_A + 1/E_B)}.$$

Thus we find $r = 0.78$ and so $\log(r) = -0.248$.

$SE(\log(r)) = 0.427$, and so an approximate 95% confidence interval for $\log(r)$ is

$$-1.10 \text{ to } 0.605$$

and so a 95% confidence interval for r is $e^{-1.10}$ to $e^{0.605}$, which is

$$0.33 \text{ to } 1.83.$$

This would imply that γ linoleic acid reduced mortality by about

119

Table 12.3   Calculation of log rank statistics for 49 patients randomly assigned to receive
γ linoleic acid (A) or control (B)

Survival time months (t_i)	Group	Total at risk (r)	Number of events (d_i)	Total at risk in group A (r_{Ai})	Expected number of events in A (E_{Ai})
0		49			
1+	A	49	0	25	0
3+	B	48	0	24	0
5+	A	47	0	24	0
6	A	46	6	23	3·0
6	A				
6	B				
6	B				
6	B				
6	B				
8	B	40	2	21	1·05
8	B				
9+	A	38	0	21	0
10	A	37	2	20	1·0811
10	A				
10+	A				
12	A	34	6	17	3·0
12	A				
12	A				
12	A				
12	B				
12	B				
12+	A				
12+	B				
13+	A	26	0	12	0
15+	A	25	0	11	0
15+	B	24	0	10	0
16+	A	23	0	10	0
16+	B	22	0	9	0
18+	B	21	0	9	0
18+	B				
20	B	19	1	9	0·4736
20+	A				
22+	B	17	0	8	0
24	A	16	2	8	1·0
24	B				
24+	A				
27+	A	13	0	6	0
28+	B	12	0	5	0
28+	B				
28+	B				
30	B	9	1	5	0·5555
30+	B				
32	A	7	1	5	0·7143
33+	B	6	0	4	0
34+	A	5	0	4	0
36+	A	4	0	3	0
36+	A				
42	B	2	1	1	0·50
44+	A				

78% compared with the control group, but with a very wide confidence interval. In view of the very small χ^2 statistic, we have little evidence that this result would not have arisen by chance.

Further methods

In the same way that multiple regression is an extension of linear regression, an extension of the log rank test includes, for example, allowance for prognostic factors. This was developed by DR Cox, and so is called *Cox regression*. It is beyond the scope of this book, but is described elsewhere.[4 5]

Common questions

Do I need to test for a constant relative risk before doing the log rank test?

This is a similar problem to testing for Normality for a t test. The log rank test is quite "robust" against departures from proportional hazards, but care should be taken. If the Kaplan–Meier survival curves cross then this is clear departure from proportional hazards, and the log rank test should not be used. This can happen, for example, in a two drug trial for cancer, if one drug is very toxic initially but produces more long term cures. In this case there is no simple answer to the question "is one drug better than the other?", because the answer depends on the time scale.

If I don't have any censored observations, do I need to use survival analysis?

Not necessarily, you could use a rank test such as the Mann–Whitney U test, but the survival method would yield an estimate of risk, which is often required, and lends itself to a useful way of displaying the data.

1 Peto R, Pike MC, Armitage P *et al*. Design and analysis of randomized clinical trials requiring prolonged observation of each patient: II. Analysis and examples. *Br J Cancer* 1977;**35**:1–39.
2 McIllmurray MB, Turkie W. Controlled trial of γ linoleic acid in Dukes' C colorectal cancer. *BMJ* 1987;**294**:1260, **295**:475.
3 Gardner MJ, Altman DG (Eds). In: *Statistics with Confidence, Confidence Intervals and Statistical Guidelines*. London: BMJ Publishing Group, 1989; Chapter 7.

4 Armitage P, Berry G. In: *Statistical Methods in Medical Practice*. Oxford: Blackwell Scientific Publications, 1994:477–81.
5 Altman DG. *Practical Statistics for Medical Research*. London: Chapman & Hall, 1991.

Exercises

Exercise 12.1

Twenty patients, ten of normal weight and ten severely overweight underwent an exercise stress test, in which they had to lift a progressively increasing load for up to 12 minutes, but they were allowed to stop earlier if they could do no more. On two occasions the equipment failed before 12 minutes. The times (in minutes) achieved were:

Normal weight: 4, 10, 12*, 2, 8, 12*, 8†, 6, 9, 12*

Overweight: 7†, 5, 11, 6, 3, 9, 4, 1, 7, 12*

*Reached end of test; †equipment failure. (I am grateful to C Osmond for these data). What are the observed and expected values? What is the value of the log rank test to compare these groups?

Exercise 12.2

What is the risk of stopping in the normal weight group compared with the overweight group, and a 95% confidence interval?

13 Study design and choosing a statistical test

Design

In many ways the design of a study is more important than the analysis. A badly designed study can never be retrieved, whereas a poorly analysed one can usually be reanalysed.[1] Consideration of design is also important because the design of a study will govern how the data are to be analysed.

Most medical studies consider an input, which may be a medical intervention or exposure to a potentially toxic compound, and an output, which is some measure of health that the intervention is supposed to affect. The simplest way to categorise studies is with reference to the time sequence in which the input and output are studied.

The most powerful studies are *prospective* studies, and the paradigm for these is the *randomised controlled* trial. In this subjects with a disease are randomised to one of two (or more) treatments, one of which may be a control treatment. Methods of randomisation have been described in Chapter 3. The importance of randomisation is that we know in the long run treatment groups will be balanced in known and *unknown* prognostic factors. It is important that the treatments are *concurrent*—that the active and control treatments occur in the same period of time.

A *parallel group* design is one in which treatment and control are allocated to different individuals. To allow for the therapeutic effect of simply being given treatment, the control may consist of a *placebo*, an inert substance that is physically identical to the active compound. If possible a study should be *double blinded*—neither the investigator nor the subject being aware of what treatment the subject is undergoing. Sometimes it is impossible to blind the subjects, for example when the treatment is some form of health education, but often it is possible to ensure that the people evaluating the outcome are unaware of the treatment. An example of a parallel group trial is given in Table 7.1, in which different bran preparations have been tested on different individuals.

A *matched* design comes about when randomisation is between matched pairs, such as in Exercise 6.2, in which randomisation was between different parts of a patient's body.

A *crossover* study is one in which two or more treatments are applied sequentially to the same subject. The advantages are that each subject then acts as their own control and so fewer subjects may be required. The main disadvantage is that there may be a carry over effect in that the action of the second treatment is affected by the first treatment. An example of a crossover trial is given in Table 7.2, in which different dosages of bran are compared within the same individual. A number of excellent books are available on clinical trials.[23]

One of the major threats to validity of a clinical trial is compliance. Patients are likely to drop out of trials if the treatment is unpleasant, and often fail to take medication as prescribed. It is usual to adopt a pragmatic approach and analyse by *intention to treat*, that is analyse the study by the treatment that the subject was assigned to, not the one they actually took. The alternative is to analyse *per protocol* or *on study*. Drop outs should of course be reported by treatment group. A checklist for writing reports on clinical trials is available.[45]

A *quasi experimental* design is one in which treatment allocation is not random. An example of this is given in Table 9.1 in which injuries are compared in two dropping zones. This is subject to potential biases in that the reason why a person is allocated to a particular dropping zone may be related to their risk of a sprained ankle.

A *cohort* study is one in which subjects, initially disease free, are followed up over a period of time. Some will be exposed to some risk factor, for example cigarette smoking. The outcome may be death and we may be interested in relating the risk factor to a particular cause of death. Clearly, these have to be large, long term studies and tend to be costly to carry out. If records have been kept routinely in the past then a historical cohort study may be carried out, an example of which is the appendicitis study discussed in Chapter 6. Here, the cohort is all cases of appendicitis admitted over a given period and a sample of the records could be inspected retrospectively. A typical example would be to look at birth weight records and relate birth weight to disease in later life.

These studies differ in essence from retrospective studies, which start with diseased subjects and then examine possible exposure. Such *case control* studies are commonly undertaken as a preliminary investigation, because they are relatively quick and inexpensive. The comparison of the blood pressure in farmers and printers given in Chapter 3 is an example of a case control study. It is retrospective because we argued from the blood pressure to the occupation and did not start out with subjects assigned to occupation. There are many confounding factors in case control studies. For example, does occupational stress cause high blood pressure, or do people prone to high blood pressure choose stressful occupations? A particular problem is recall bias, in that the cases, with the disease, are more motivated to recall apparently trivial episodes in the past than controls, who are disease free.

Cross sectional studies are common and include surveys, laboratory experiments and studies to examine the prevalence of a disease. Studies validating instruments and questionnaires are also cross sectional studies. The study of urinary concentration of lead in children described in Chapter 1 and the study of the relationship between height and pulmonary anatomical dead space in Chapter 11 were also cross sectional studies.

Sample size

One of the most common questions asked of a statistician about design is the number of patients to include. It is an important question, because if a study is too small it will not be able to answer the question posed, and would be a waste of time and money. It could also be deemed unethical because patients may be put at risk with no apparent benefit. However, studies should not be too large because resources would be wasted if fewer patients would have sufficed. The sample size depends on four critical quantities: the type I and type II error rates α and β (discussed in Chapter 5), the variability of the data σ^2, and the effect size d. In a trial the effect size is the amount by which we would expect the two treatments to differ, or is the difference that would be clinically worthwhile.

Usually α and β are fixed at 5% and 20% (or 10%) respectively. A simple formula for a two group parallel trial with a continuous outcome is that the required sample size per group is given by n = $16\sigma^2/d^2$ for two sided α of 5% and β of 20%. For example, in a trial to reduce blood pressure, if a clinically worthwhile effect for diastolic blood pressure is 5 mmHg and the between subjects standard deviation is 10 mmHg, we would require n = 16 × 100/25 = 64 patients per group in the study. The sample size goes up as the square of the standard deviation of the data (the variance) and goes down inversely as the square of the effect size. Doubling the effect size reduces the sample size by four—it is much easier to detect large effects! In practice, the sample size is often fixed by other criteria, such as finance or resources, and the formula is used to determine a realistic effect size. If this is too large, then the study will have to be abandoned or increased in size. Machin *et al.* give advice on a sample size calculations for a wide variety of study designs.[6]

Choice of test

In terms of selecting a statistical test, the most important question is "what is the main study hypothesis?" In some cases there is no hypothesis; the investigator just wants to "see what is there". For example, in a prevalence study there is no hypothesis to test, and the size of the study is determined by how accurately the investigator wants to determine the prevalence. If there is no hypothesis, then there is no statistical test. It is important to decide *a priori* which hypotheses are confirmatory (that is, are testing some presupposed relationship), and which are exploratory (are suggested by the data). No single study can support a whole series of hypotheses.

126

A sensible plan is to limit severely the number of confirmatory hypotheses. Although it is valid to use statistical tests on hypotheses suggested by the data, the P values should be used only as guidelines, and the results treated as very tentative until confirmed by subsequent studies. A useful guide is to use a *Bonferroni* correction, which states simply that if one is testing n independent hypotheses, one should use a significance level of $0.05/n$. Thus if there were two independent hypotheses a result would be declared significant only if $P<0.025$. Note that, since tests are rarely independent, this is a very conservative procedure—one unlikely to reject the null hypothesis.

The investigator should then ask "are the data independent?" This can be difficult to decide but as a rule of thumb results on the same individual, or from matched individuals, are not independent. Thus results from a crossover trial, or from a case control study in which the controls were matched to the cases by age, sex and social class, are not independent. It is generally true that the analysis should reflect the design, and so a matched design should be followed by a matched analysis. Results measured over time require special care.[7] One of the most common mistakes in statistical analysis is to treat dependent variables as independent. For example, suppose we were looking at treatment of leg ulcers, in which some people had an ulcer on each leg. We might have 20 subjects with 30 ulcers but the number of independent pieces of information is 20 because the state of an ulcer on one leg may influence the state of the ulcer on the other leg and an analysis that considered ulcers as independent observations would be incorrect. For a correct analysis of mixed paired and unpaired data consult a statistician.

The next question is "what types of data are being measured?" The test used should be determined by the data. The choice of test for matched or paired data is described in Table 13.1 and for independent data in Table 13.2.

It is helpful to decide the *input* variables and the *outcome* variables. For example in a clinical trial the input variable is type of treatment—a nominal variable—and the outcome may be some clinical measure—perhaps Normally distributed. The required test is then the *t* test (Table 13.2). However, if the input variable is continuous, say a clinical score, and the outcome is nominal, say cured or not cured, logistic regression is the required analysis. A *t*

127

Table 13.1   *Choice of statistical test from paired or matched observations*

Variable	Test
Nominal	McNemar's Test
Ordinal (Ordered categories)	Wilcoxon
Quantitative (Discrete or Non-Normal)	Wilcoxon
Quantitative (Normal*)	Paired t test

* It is the *difference* between the paired observations that should be plausibly Normal.

test in this case may help but would not give us what we require, namely the probability of a cure for a given value of the clinical score. As another example, suppose we have a cross sectional study in which we ask a random sample of people whether they think their general practitioner is doing a good job, on a five point scale, and we wish to ascertain whether women have a higher opinion of general practitioners than men have. The input variable is gender, which is nominal. The outcome variable is the five point ordinal scale. Each person's opinion is independent of the others, so we have independent data. From Table 13.2 we should use a χ^2 test for trend, or a Mann–Whitney U test (with correction for ties). Note, however, if some people share a general practitioner and others do not, then the data are not independent and a more sophisticated analysis is called for.

Note that these tables should be considered as guides only, and each case should be considered on its merits.

1 Campbell MJ, Machin D. In: *Medical Statistics: A Common-sense Approach*, 2nd edn. Chichester: Wiley, 1993:2.
2 Pocock SJ. *Clinical trials: A Practical Approach.* Chichester: Wiley, 1982.
3 Senn SJ. *The Design and Analysis of Cross-Over Trials.* Chichester: Wiley, 1992.
4 Gardner MJ, Altman DG (eds) In: *Statistics with Confidence.* BMJ Publishing Group, 1989: 103–5.
5 Gardner MJ, Machin D, Campbell MJ. The use of checklists in assessing the statistical content of medical studies. *BMJ* 1986;**292**:810–12.
6 Machin D, Campbell MJ, Fayers P, Pinol A. *Statistical Tables for the Design of Clinical Studies.* Oxford: Blackwell Scientific Publications, 1996.
7 Matthews JNS, Altman DG, Campbell MJ, Royston JP. Analysis of serial measurements in medical research. *BMJ* 1990;**300**:230–5.
8 Altman DG. *Practical Statistics for Medical Research.* London: Chapman & Hall, 1991.
9 Armitage P, Berry G. In: *Statistical Methods in Medical Research.* Oxford: Blackwell Scientific Publications, 1994.

Table 13.2 Choice of statistical test for independent observations

		Outcome variable				
		Nominal	Categorical (>2 Categories)	Ordinal	Quantitative Discrete	Quantitative Non-Normal	Quantitative Normal
Input Variable	Nominal	χ² or Fisher's	χ²	χ²-trend or Mann–Whitney	Mann–Whitney	Mann–Whitney or log-rank[a]	Student's t test
	Categorical (>2 categories)	χ²	χ²	Kruskal–Wallis[b]	Kruskal–Wallis[b]	Kruskal–Wallis[b]	Analysis of variance[c]
	Ordinal (Ordered categories)	χ²-trend or Mann–Whitney	[e]	Spearman rank	Spearman rank	Spearman rank	Spearman rank or linear regression[d]
	Quantitative Discrete	Logistic regression	[e]	[e]	Spearman rank	Spearman rank	Spearman rank or linear regression[d]
	Quantitative non-Normal	Logistic regression	[e]	[e]	[e]	Plot data and Pearson or Spearman rank	Plot data and Pearson or Spearman rank and linear regression
	Quantitative Normal	Logistic regression	[e]	[e]	[e]	Linear regression[d]	Pearson and linear regression

[a] If data are censored.

[b] The Kruskal–Wallis test is used for comparing ordinal or non-Normal variables for more than two groups, and is a generalisation of the Mann–Whitney U test. The technique is beyond the scope of this book, but is described in more advanced books[8,9] and is available in common software (Epi-Info, Minitab, SPSS).

[c] Analysis of variance is a general technique, and one version (one way analysis of variance) is used to compare Normally distributed variables for more than two groups, and is the parametric equivalent of the Kruskal–Wallis test.

[d] If the outcome variable is the *dependent* variable, then provided the residuals (see Chapter 11) are plausibly Normal, then the distribution of the independent variable is not important.

[e] There are a number of more advanced techniques, such as Poisson regression, for dealing with these situations. However, they require certain assumptions and it is often easier to either dichotomise the outcome variable or treat it as continuous.

Exercises

State the type of study described in each of the following.

Exercise 13.1

To investigate the relationship between egg consumption and heart disease, a group of patients admitted to hospital with myocardial infarction were questioned about their egg consumption. A group of age and sex matched patients admitted to a fracture clinic were also questioned about their egg consumption using an identical protocol.

Exercise 13.2

To investigate the relationship between certain solvents and cancer, all employees at a factory were questioned about their exposure to an industrial solvent, and the amount and length of exposure measured. These subjects were regularly monitored, and after 10 years a copy of the death certificate for all those who had died was obtained.

Exercise 13.3

A survey was conducted of all nurses employed at a particular hospital. Among other questions, the questionnaire asked about the grade of the nurse and whether she was satisfied with her career prospects.

Exercise 13.4

To evaluate a new back school, patients with lower back pain were randomly allocated to either the new school or to conventional occupational therapy. After 3 months they were questioned about their back pain, and observed lifting a weight by independent monitors.

Exercise 13.5

A new triage system has been set up at the local Accident and Emergency Unit. To evaluate it the waiting times of patients were measured for 6 months and compared with the waiting times at a comparable nearby hospital.

Answers to exercises

1.1 Median 0·71, range 0·10 to 1·24, first quartile 0·535, third quartile 0·84 μmol/24h.

2.1 Mean = 2·41, SD = 1·27.

2.2 Mean = 0·697 μmol/24h, SD = 0·2410 μmol/24h, range 0·215 to 1·179 μmol/l.

2.3 Points 0·10 and 1·24. 2/40 or 5%.

3.1 SE(mean) = 0·074 μmol/24 h.

3.2 A uniform or flat distribution. Population mean 4·5, population SD 2·87.

3.3 The distribution will be approximately Normal, mean 4·5 and SD $2·87/\sqrt{5} = 1·28$.

4.1 The reference range is 12·26–57·74, and so the observed value of 52 is included in it.

4.2 95% CI 32·73 to 37·27.

5.1 0·42 g/dl, $z = 3·08$ $0·001 < P < 0·01$, difference = 1·3 g/dl, 95% CI 0·48 to 2·12 g/dl.

5.2 0·23 g/dl, P < 0·001.

6.1 SE (percentage) = 2·1%, SE (difference) = 3·7%, difference = 3·4%. 95% CI −3·9 to 10·7%, $z = 0·94$, P = 0·35.

6.2 Yes, the traditional remedy, $z = 2·2$, P = 0·028.

7.1 37·5 to 40·5 KA units.

7.2 $t = 2·652$, d.f. = 17, $0·01 < P < 0·02$.

7.3 0·56 g/dl, t = 1·243, d.f. = 20, 0·1<P<0·5, 95% CI −0·38 to 1·50 g/dl.

7.4 15 days, t = 1·758, d.f. = 9, 0·1<P<0·5, 95% CI −4·30 to 34·30 days.

8.1 Standard $\chi^2 = 3·295$, d.f. = 4, P>0·5. Trend $\chi^2 = 2·25$, d.f. = 1, P = 0·13.

8.2 $X^2 = 3·916$, d.f. = 1, 0·02<P<0·05, difference in rates 9%, 95% CI 0·3 to 17·9%.

8.3 $X^2 = 0·931$, d.f. = 1, 0·1<P<0·5, difference in rates 15%, 95% CI −7·7 to 38%.

8.4 $X^2 = 8·949$, d.f. = 3, 0·02<P<0·05. Yes, practice C; if this is omitted the remaining practices give $X^2 = 0·241$, d.f. = 2, P>0·5. (Both χ^2 tests by quick method.)

9.1 Sickness rate in first department = 28%, in second department 8%, difference 20% (approximate 95% CI = −6 to 45%, P = 0·24 (Fisher's Exact test mid P)). P is calculated from $2 \times (0·5 \times 0·173 + 0·031)$.

10.1 Smaller total = −30. No.

10.2 Mann–Whitney statistic = 74. The group on the new remedy. No.

11.1 r = −0·848.

11.2 rs = −0·867.

11.3 y = 36·1 − 2·34x. This means that, on average, for every 1 mile increase in mean distance the attendance rate drops by 2·34%. This can be safely accepted only within the area measured here.

11.4 SE = 0·39, 95% CI = −2·34 − 2·145 × 0·39 to −2·34 + 2·145 × 0·39 = −3·1 to −1·5%.

12.1 $O_A = 6$, $t_A = 8·06$, $O_B = 8$, $E_B = 5·94$. Log rank $X^2 = 1·24$, d.f. = 1, 0·1<P<0·5.

12.2 Risk = 0·55, 95% CI 0·19 to 1·60.

13.1 Matched case control study.

13.2 Cohort study.

13.3 Cross sectional study.

13.4 Randomised controlled trial.

13.5 Quasi experimental design.

Appendix

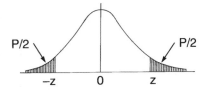

Table A   Probabilities related to multiples of standard deviations for a Normal distribution

Number of standard deviations (z)	Probability of getting an observation at least as far from the mean (two sided P)
0·0	1·00
0·1	0·92
0·2	0·84
0·3	0·76
0·4	0·69
0·5	0·62
0·6	0·55
0·674	0·500
0·7	0·48
0·8	0·42
0·9	0·37
1·0	0·31
1·1	0·27
1·2	0·23
1·3	0·19
1·4	0·16
1·5	0·13
1·6	0·11
1·645	0·100
1·7	0·089
1·8	0·072
1·9	0·057
1·96	0·050
2·0	0·045
2·1	0·036
2·2	0·028
2·3	0·021
2·4	0·016
2·5	0·012
2·576	0·010
3·0	0·0027
3·291	0·0010

Table B   Distribution of t *(two tailed)*

	Probability					
d.f.	0·5	0·1	0·05	0·02	0·01	0·001
1	1·000	6·314	12·706	31·821	63·657	636·619
2	0·816	2·920	4·303	6·965	9·925	31·598
3	0·765	2·353	3·182	4·541	5·841	12·941
4	0·741	2·132	2·776	3·747	4·604	8·610
5	0·727	2·015	2·571	3·365	4·032	6·859
6	0·718	1·943	2·447	3·143	3·707	5·959
7	0·711	1·895	2·365	2·998	3·499	5·405
8	0·706	1·860	2·306	2·896	3·355	5·041
9	0·703	1·833	2·262	2·821	3·250	4·781
10	0·700	1·812	2·228	2·764	3·169	4·587
11	0·697	1·796	2·201	2·718	3·106	4·437
12	0·695	1·782	2·179	2·681	3·055	4·318
13	0·694	1·771	2·160	2·650	3·012	4·221
14	0·692	1·761	2·145	2·624	2·977	4·140
15	0·691	1·753	2·131	2·602	2·947	4·073
16	0·690	1·746	2·120	2·583	2·921	4·015
17	0·689	1·740	2·110	2·567	2·898	3·965
18	0·688	1·734	2·101	2·552	2·878	3·922
19	0·688	1·729	2·093	2·539	2·861	3·883
20	0·687	1·725	2·086	2·528	2·845	3·850
21	0·686	1·721	2·080	2·518	2·831	3·819
22	0·686	1·717	2·074	2·508	2·819	3·792
23	0·685	1·714	2·069	2·500	2·807	3·767
24	0·685	1·711	2·064	2·492	2·797	3·745
25	0·684	1·708	2·060	2·485	2·787	3·725
26	0·684	1·706	2·056	2·479	2·779	3·707
27	0·684	1·703	2·052	2·473	2·771	3·690
28	0·683	1·701	2·048	2·467	2·763	3·674
29	0·683	1·699	2·045	2·462	2·756	3·659
30	0·683	1·697	2·042	2·457	2·750	3·646
40	0·681	1·684	2·021	2·423	2·704	3·551
60	0·679	1·671	2·000	2·390	2·660	3·460
120	0·677	1·658	1·980	2·358	2·617	3·373
∞	0·674	1·645	1·960	2·326	2·576	3·291

Adapted by permission of the authors and publishers from Table III of Fisher and Yates: *Statistical Tables for Biological, Agricultural and Medical Research*, published by Longman Group Ltd., London (previously published by Oliver & Boyd, Edinburgh).

Table C   Distribution of χ^2

d.f.	Probability					
	0·50	0·10	0·05	0·02	0·01	0·001
1	0·455	2·706	3·841	5·412	6·635	10·827
2	1·386	4·605	5·991	7·824	9·210	13·815
3	2·366	6·251	7·815	9·837	11·345	16·268
4	3·357	7·779	9·488	11·668	13·277	18·465
5	4·351	9·236	11·070	13·388	15·086	20·517
6	5·348	10·645	12·592	15·033	16·812	22·457
7	6·346	12·017	14·067	16·622	18·475	24·322
8	7·344	13·362	15·507	18·168	20·090	26·125
9	8·343	14·684	16·919	19·679	21·666	27·877
10	9·342	15·987	18·307	21·161	23·209	29·588
11	10·341	17·275	19·675	22·618	24·725	31·264
12	11·340	18·549	21·026	24·054	26·217	32·909
13	12·340	19·812	22·362	25·472	27·688	34·528
14	13·339	21·064	23·685	26·873	29·141	36·123
15	14·339	22·307	24·996	28·259	30·578	37·697
16	15·338	23·542	26·296	29·633	32·000	39·252
17	16·338	24·769	27·587	30·995	33·409	40·790
18	17·338	25·989	28·869	32·346	34·805	42·312
19	18·338	27·204	30·144	33·687	36·191	43·820
20	19·337	28·412	31·410	35·020	37·566	45·315
21	20·337	29·615	32·671	36·343	38·932	46·797
22	21·337	30·813	33·924	37·659	40·289	48·268
23	22·337	32·007	35·172	38·968	41·638	49·728
24	23·337	33·196	36·415	40·270	42·980	51·179
25	24·337	34·382	37·652	41·566	44·314	52·620
26	25·336	35·563	38·885	42·856	45·642	54·052
27	26·336	36·741	40·113	44·140	46·963	55·476
28	27·336	37·916	41·337	45·419	48·278	56·893
29	28·336	39·087	42·557	46·693	49·588	58·302
30	29·336	40·256	43·773	47·962	50·892	59·703

Adapted by permission of the authors and publishers from Table IV of Fisher and Yates, *Statistical Tables for Biological, Agricultural and Medical Research*, published by Longman Group Ltd., London (previously published by Oliver & Boyd, Edinburgh).

Table D   Wilcoxon test on paired samples: 5% and 1% levels of P

Number of pairs	5% Level	1% Level
7	2	0
8	2	0
9	6	2
10	8	3
11	11	5
12	14	7
13	17	10
14	21	13
15	25	16
16	30	19

Reprinted (slightly abbreviated) by permission of the publisher from *Statistical Methods*, 6th edition, by George W Snedecor and William G Cochran (copyright), 1967, Iowa State University Press, Ames, Iowa, USA.

Table E   Mann–Whitney test on unpaired samples: 5% and 1% levels of P

5% Critical points of rank sums

n_2 ↓ \ n_1 →	2	3	4	5	6	7	8	9	10	11	12	13	14	15
4			10											
5		6	11	17										
6		7	12	18	26									
7		7	13	20	27	36								
8	3	8	14	21	29	38	49							
9	3	8	15	22	31	40	51	63						
10	3	9	15	23	32	42	53	65	78					
11	4	9	16	24	34	44	55	68	81	96				
12	4	10	17	26	35	46	58	71	85	99	115			
13	4	10	18	27	37	48	60	73	88	103	119	137		
14	4	11	19	28	38	50	63	76	91	106	123	141	160	
15	4	11	20	29	40	52	65	79	94	110	127	145	164	185
16	4	12	21	31	42	54	67	82	97	114	131	150	169	
17	5	12	21	32	43	56	70	84	100	117	135	154		
18	5	13	22	33	45	58	72	87	103	121	139			
19	5	13	23	34	46	60	74	90	107	124				
20	5	14	24	35	48	62	77	93	110					
21	6	14	25	37	50	64	79	95						
22	6	15	26	38	51	66	82							
23	6	15	27	39	53	68								
24	6	16	28	40	55									
25	6	16	28	42										
26	7	17	29											
27	7	17												
28	7													

1% Critical points of rank sums

n₂ ↓ \ n₁ →	2	3	4	5	6	7	8	9	10	11	12	13	14	15
5				15										
6			10	16	23									
7			10	17	24	32								
8			11	17	25	34	43							
9		6	11	18	26	35	45	56						
10		6	12	19	27	37	47	58	71					
11		6	12	20	28	38	49	61	74	87				
12		7	13	21	30	40	51	63	76	90	106			
13		7	14	22	31	41	53	65	79	93	109	125		
14		7	14	22	32	43	54	67	81	96	112	129	147	
15		8	15	23	33	44	56	70	84	99	115	133	151	171
16		8	15	24	34	46	58	72	86	102	119	137	155	
17		8	16	25	36	47	60	74	89	105	122	140		
18		8	16	26	37	49	62	76	92	108	125			
19	3	9	17	27	38	50	64	78	94	111				
20	3	9	18	28	39	52	66	81	97					
21	3	9	18	29	40	53	68	83						
22	3	10	19	29	42	55	70							
23	3	10	19	30	43	57								
24	3	10	20	31	44									
25	3	11	20	32										
26	3	11	21											
27	4	11												
28	4													

n_1 and n_2 are the numbers of cases in the two groups. If the groups are unequal in size, n_1 refers to the smaller.

Reproduced by permission of the author and publisher from White C, *Biometrics* 1952;8:33.

Table F   Random numbers

```
35368 65415 14425 97294 44734 54870 84495 39332 72708 52000 02219 86130 30264 56203 26518
93023 53965 19527 72819 42973 38037 37056 13200 09831 41367 40828 25938 05655 99010 88115
92226 65530 10966 29733 73902 19009 74733 68041 83166 92796 64846 79200 38776 09312 72234
15542 85361 44069 61445 82994 45169 79458 52221 37132 67125 62700 83475 99850 31670 50750
96424 65745 74877 48473 54281 67837 11167 74898 83136 10498 10660 65810 16373 80382 21874
17946 97751 54049 83077 03256 51947 88278 23891 53495 07101 95811 73035 83017 18532 59650
71495 36712 01513 30802 47228 52799 97961 82519 22756 69151 09052 38681 38858 38807 02422
16762 98574 78301 62647 29247 22936 62778 56694 70597 48880 33162 76138 97425 78283 42063
37969 66660 77823 54923 75832 99974 13868 94446 99521 44775 76649 00502 73424 21068 87880
25471 88920 39906 81436 70910 02631 93238 41952 87493 33559 64733 24688 78583 31506 24845
68507 79643 15204 84794 60093 29874 61851 05751 21960 70131 42137 73723 19252 23912 77751
67385 88293 46249 53036 47309 68803 15155 28222 06764 92367 25490 18494 42546 75268 05988
58948 40572 79817 40486 40494 20843 07388 74732 71655 17445 28489 84528 93922 67324 59120
70476 23299 17965 93629 28988 82399 81811 86373 91600 99962 28784 77326 24912 81992 66011
72887 41730 95940 54210 58480 96724 41954 91803 43078 85644 50014 93038 56037 79787 10707
70205 26256 91417 78629 16268 47156 32065 54588 74250 24739 04128 53966 74106 70159 80428
78883 36361 28182 51842 61426 27799 75951 58854 77236 04606 26949 56428 28495 41766 50059
89970 55101 66660 36953 02774 45020 54998 19226 44811 96941 70693 68847 07633 22289 94290
34382 04274 02116 37857 72075 90908 56584 67907 15075 63216 49006 24748 34289 55142 91206
16999 91140 64818 23018 09217 46068 32467 63844 72589 35456 44840 90800 50692 33298 74323
16329 39676 37510 35590 45888 77371 58301 79434 17500 48320 08953 18242 15133 24137 07323
31983 83436 93006 12640 00403 91457 62602 12245 27670 61492 89166 69421 79505 47104 50817
92780 80153 81458 82215 71536 03586 44007 85679 68186 85375 15373 57441 10034 74455 18466
70834 75678 78777 79731 06046 02386 18059 89623 65480 69345 49447 10358 74307 68861 87853
10100 85365 77687 36241 87563 06298 81828 40194 30647 36237 17793 50680 63701 39522 86006
84265 60501 17148 13657 40775 64773 62103 16356 99405 00598 81881 62732 36765 11895 63933
74041 62109 30831 62133 29462 30144 62081 79158 09737 72614 74806 25554 50911 43289 30344
02882 45141 58967 19688 48208 65679 18296 19080 03529 46017 33799 45518 31075 39740 93387
67647 56443 57816 49471 23525 76582 30085 90312 07397 42747 04242 58569 80087 45598 34374
99668 68326 47357 94812 65654 01097 55260 80990 46748 06416 93919 64520 54666 82278 59328
12013 30983 00370 40243 44457 18279 69740 39061 00548 21321 11249 48478 14917 26056 89506
55581 69068 66561 75671 07363 22939 93007 45319 48358 27534 60873 51076 20823 28185 49038
74957 53949 40414 15035 90232 28946 78073 75923 43081 16030 32935 30947 64395 03271 21345
65073 60950 92314 02037 82817 33518 49680 20095 51301 91889 78488 75298 29067 11355 69994
05110 83292 51335 64460 37648 72915 99688 62628 41297 36039 04436 82738 76614 55630 35803
54053 98104 12386 15646 89759 55889 14513 96192 19957 06186 40853 38011 97401 04047 66722
52351 72086 70257 83693 62924 79060 79683 03143 10627 45371 78404 50185 67515 65094 91111
10759 18901 07590 07727 37140 95782 41994 71688 72341 73665 66833 14138 20949 91852 42847
67322 87517 27043 12936 81043 27338 81679 88420 28220 65441 55517 96640 60178 84161 64239
37634 07842 34936 26836 48230 52786 01114 61335 39149 34268 70089 93491 91616 22522 06577
90556 62996 52252 42541 12781 40917 41661 96994 88818 93137 45130 34502 40479 65832 79294
07067 12854 23166 49012 56479 22674 69603 47846 91920 19188 94206 30370 50741 79932 88916
82945 28472 46267 45857 67101 39905 25753 75462 87523 01394 10135 26758 88652 34480 37901
33399 81517 64127 82407 23689 46598 23814 89327 87057 67715 30785 58496 38661 23259 19631
51428 25572 62696 33117 66242 11735 68466 90598 30201 25770 96006 48256 60967 49546 74989
45246 23347 48896 15828 69240 93948 27855 21999 19155 72859 78754 40094 39323 37570 73953
24384 49141 78464 73448 78883 25730 24813 36087 47883 50473 38354 25620 08787 61463 95219
43550 53461 42673 12646 87988 01411 58160 76833 53423 45490 23316 84940 81917 52712 10575
67691 02660 28326 46648 00840 02753 12403 29024 03017 28175 23557 64382 71324 17581 63090
49360 13426 04763 85671 40498 18689 99523 50400 00562 02112 00219 84376 42585 90350 96349
42432 49348 10219 99564 70165 82692 85914 81874 60401 37323 80781 59989 00844 82734 60942
68547 85157 26956 52508 10019 18964 03084 21624 95686 76579 53032 44148 74984 81609 42544
26081 21040 57502 30827 61940 50305 13410 22158 91529 35888 48318 13355 12491 31827 31256
16113 01090 72822 51906 23547 06985 93466 74652 33329 18298 75319 55988 76412 47573 49236
88368 50633 62276 50244 14896 21158 49633 92045 25400 49228 20287 69106 32732 88075 20196
37861 95795 39254 87408 16929 87171 38600 61330 80663 56488 43425 08589 53842 39410 55751
```

Index

139

Related titles

STATISTICS IN CLINICAL PRACTICE

David Coggon

This concise text explains the principles of statistics for anyone needing to understand them in the journals and in clinical practice. Three sections include: summarising data numerically and graphically; the concept of probability; and methods of drawing conclusions from observation made on samples of patients or clinical therapeutics. Illustrated with clinical examples throughout, and test questions at the end of each section, this is the ideal introduction for all clinicians.

Readership: all medical staff, medical students

MEDICAL STATISTICS ON PERSONAL COMPUTERS *Second edition*

R A Brown, J Swanson Beck

This book shows how to get the best out of the software available for analysing statistical data on personal computers. This completely revised second edition includes new chapters on survival analysis, statistical power calculations, writing up statistical analyses for medical papers, and useful notes on packages available – making it a thoroughly practical guide.

Readership: medical researchers, clinicians doing medical research

EPIDEMIOLOGY FOR THE UNINITIATED

Third edition

Geoffrey Rose, D J P Barker, D Coggon

In this well established and popular introduction, the novice is expertly guided through the theory and practical pitfalls of epidemiological study. The third edition contains new sections on randomised controlled trials and on reading and interpreting epidemiological reports.

Readership: students, GPs, medical researchers

For further details contact your local bookseller, or in case of difficulty, contact the Books Division, BMJ Publishing Group, BMA House, Tavistock Square, London WC1H 9JR, UK (Tel +44(0) 171-383-6245; Fax: +44(0) 171-383 6662)